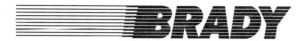

Communicable Diseases and Infection Control for EMS

Robert G. Nixon, BA, EMT-P

Brady/Prentice Hall Health
Upper Saddle River, New Jersey 07458

Library of Congress Cataloging-in-Publication Data

Nixon, Robert G.
    Communicable diseases and infection control for EMS / Robert G. Nixon.
      p.   cm.
    Includes index.
    ISBN 0-13-084384-9 (paper)
    1. Emergency medical technicians—Health and hygiene.   2. Emergency
medicine—Safety measures.   3. Infections—Prevention.   4. Communicable
diseases—Prevention.   I. Title.
    RC965.E48 N55 2000
    616.9′045—dc21
                                        99-044939
                                          CIP

PUBLISHER: *Julie Alexander*
ACQUISITIONS EDITOR: *Judy Streger*
EDITORIAL ASSISTANT: *Jeanne Molenaar*
DIRECTOR OF PRODUCTION AND MANUFACTURING: *Bruce Johnson*
MANAGING PRODUCTION EDITOR: *Patrick Walsh*
SENIOR PRODUCTION MANAGER: *Ilene Sanford*
PRODUCTION EDITOR: *Danielle Newhouse*
CREATIVE DIRECTOR: *Marianne Frasco*
INTERIOR DESIGNERS: *Julie Boddorf/Danielle Newhouse*
COVER DESIGNER: *Maria Guglielmo*
COVER PHOTO: *Photo Researchers Inc/Science Source*
MARKETING MANAGER: *Tiffany Price*
MARKETING COORDINATOR: *Cindy Frederick*
COMPOSITION: *Rainbow Graphics, LLC*
PRINTING AND BINDING: *The Banta Company*

© 2000 by Prentice-Hall, Inc.
Upper Saddle River, New Jersey 07458

Printed in the United States of America

10 9 8 7 6 5 4 3 2 1

ISBN 0-13-084384-9

PRENTICE-HALL INTERNATIONAL (UK) LIMITED, *London*
PRENTICE-HALL OF AUSTRALIA PTY. LIMITED, *Sydney*
PRENTICE-HALL CANADA, INC., *Toronto*
PRENTICE-HALL HISPANOAMERICANA, S.A., *Mexico*
PRENTICE-HALL OF INDIA PRIVATE LIMITED, *New Delhi*
PRENTICE-HALL OF JAPAN, INC., *Tokyo*
PRENTICE-HALL SINGAPORE PTE. LTD.
EDITORA PRENTICE-HALL DO BRASIL, LTDA., *Rio de Janeiro*

Contents

Preface

In the early to mid-1980s, EMS professionals became acutely aware of the risks from unseen threats faced every day. Although they were aware of the risk of injuries from improper lifting, exposed metal and glass at motor vehicle crashes, and random acts of violence, what was not considered, at least not seriously, were the threats from communicable diseases. What attracted our attention was the media's fervor over HIV and AIDS. The news media gave daily doses of information about a deadly virus spreading throughout the world, unchecked and incurable.

Since that time, federal, state, and local government agencies have mandated training in bloodborne pathogens, the use of personal protective equipment, and the implementation of infection control programs specifically targeted to reduce the chance of exposure to HIV and to lessen the chances of contracting hepatitis B. Sadly, those are not the only two diseases that we are at risk for contracting. A myriad of other illnesses—bloodborne and airborne—can infect us when we are least prepared. Some of these illnesses can be fatal or can lead to long-term disability.

This text provides concise information that can be used to guide the EMT or paramedic through the jungle of infectious diseases. Although many people have developed an immunity to some of the diseases discussed here, several illnesses still pose a risk for contracting.

The chapters are divided into several key components that are easy to read and understand. In the chapters discussing the various communicable diseases, each illness has information presented in the same sequence. For each disease, information is given on *Nature and Spread of the Disease, Signs and Symptoms,* and *Personal Protection.*

The diseases and personal protection standards described may affect EMTs and paramedics equally. Some skills may be mentioned that are performed only at the paramedic or advanced levels of certification. However, universal precautions do pertain equally to EMTs as well as paramedics.

Here is a summary of the chapters in this textbook:

CHAPTER 1: IN THE BEGINNING

This chapter addresses recognizing and combating infectious diseases. It takes a look at the role and responsibilities of the regulatory agencies such as the Centers for Disease Control and Prevention and the Occupational Health and

Safety Administration. It also discusses the chain or links necessary to cause an infection. The types of infectious agents such as bacteria, viruses, and fungi are presented. Finally, the chapter discusses the general signs and symptoms of an infectious person.

CHAPTER 2: GOING MY WAY?

Not all infectious patients will transmit the disease. This chapter focuses on how diseases are transmitted from one person to another and offers some general ideas for personal protection against contamination.

CHAPTER 3: CATCH AS CATCH CAN'T!

Why is it that when you are around someone who has an infectious disease you do not come down with it? The most likely reason is that the body's natural defenses have blocked or destroyed the invading organisms. This chapter addresses the body's natural defenses and the immune system's protection against infectious agents.

CHAPTER 4: OUT OF THE MOUTHS OF BABES

Children often contract all kinds of infectious diseases. This chapter discusses the various childhood diseases, their signs and symptoms, and how the illnesses are spread. It also suggests ways to protect against the more common childhood maladies.

CHAPTER 5: COMING OF AGE

Many diseases affect adults or are more commonly found in adulthood. This chapter presents information about illnesses typically seen in the adult population.

CHAPTER 6: WHEN THE FOOD COMES BACK TO BITE YOU!

Food poisoning is a very unpleasant experience. Although food poisoning is not typically transmitted from person to person, EMS professionals see patients with food poisoning or may come in contact with contaminated food. Common infectious agents in food are presented along with signs and symptoms of the illness they produce.

CHAPTER 7: DANGEROUS ACRONYMS

On almost everyone's mind is HIV infection and AIDS. This chapter focuses on this deadly virus and the effects of HIV infection.

CHAPTER 8: WITH A JAUNDICED EYE

Of equal if not more significance to the EMS professional is hepatitis. The hepatitis virus is much easier to transmit than HIV. This chapter addresses the various strains of hepatitis virus including A, B, C, D, E, F, and G.

CHAPTER 9: PUTTING IT ALL TOGETHER

Does your EMS agency have an Infection Control Program? Is the program effective in reducing the chance of exposure to an infectious agent? What are the steps taken after an exposure? Every EMS agency is required to have an Infection Control Program. A sample program that may be adapted to your EMS agency can be found in the Appendix.

UNIQUE FEATURES

You Make the Call

Along with chapter information, "case histories" or scenarios are presented in which you, as the EMT, are on the scene. After reading a brief description of the situation, there are questions to test your knowledge. Answers to You Make the Call are located in the Appendix.

Glossary

Each chapter contains a highlighted section of terms used in the text along with their definitions. Rather than turning to the end of the book to look up a term, refer to this glossary as the chapter is read.

It is hoped that a lot of the information in this text will be beneficial and that you become more familiar with the risks faced each time you respond to a call for help. More importantly, the major goal of this text is to help keep you safe. Be careful out there!

Acknowledgments

Nearly every book has people who work behind the scenes to get the text to its final stages and into print. *Communicable Diseases and Infection Control for EMS* is no exception. With the hard work and contributions of many people working in the background, this text has become a reality. To them, I owe a debt of gratitude and would like to recognize them now.

Thanks to Judy Streger at Brady for believing in the book and pushing me to make deadlines, some of which were, unfortunately, delayed. While Judy has moved into sales from her position as acquisition editor, her support and friendship are still felt and appreciated.

Thanks also go to Julie Pophal of Transcription Plus in Madison Wisconsin. Julie tirelessly proofread the initial drafts of the manuscript and gave me some helpful hints to make it more coherent and easier to understand.

Along with Julie, there were the reviewers whose suggestions and tips were much appreciated. Many of their suggestions for additional material were incorporated in the final work.

Harvey B. Craven
EMS Medical Control Manager
Polk County EMS
Bartow, FL

Jon R. Donnelly
Executive Director
Old Dominion EMS Alliance
Richmond, VA

Rudy Garrett
Paramedic Training Coordinator
Somerset-Pulaski Co. EMS
Somerset, KY

Marie S. Gospodareck, BS, EMT-P, MAEd
Assistant Professor, Dept of Medicine
EMS Program Director
University of Alabama at Birmingham
Birmingham, AL

Donald Graesser
Assistant Director
Bergen County EMS Training Center
Paramus, NJ

Larry J. Hill
President
Environmental, Health, Safety, and Training Consultants
Naples, FL

Erik J. Hollick, EMT-B, EMT-I/C
Hudson, MA

Louis A. Jenkins
Cleveland County EMS
Shelby, NC

Gregory Juersivich
Chief, North Canton EMS
Instructor, Stark State College
North Canton, OH

Shelby Louden, BS, EMT-P
Public Safety Services Coordinator
D. Russel Lee Career Center
Hamilton, OH

Robert McMahon
Fire and EMS Coordinator
Putnam County Bureau of Fire and
   EMS
Carmel, NY

James B. Miller, EMT-P
EMS Coordinator
Fire and Emergency Services
Fort Sam Houston, TX

Mark Monroe, BA, RN, EMT-P, MS
EMS Manager
Reichhold Inc
Valley Park, MO

William A. Moreau, NREMT-P,
   EMT-I/C
ASCJ
Florida, MA

Virginia K. Riedy
Program Director
Medical College of Ohio
Toledo, OH

I would also like to thank Brooke Hastings who appears in some of the photographs wearing or demonstrating some of the personal protective equipment.

Jacob Kipp also deserves my thanks for contributing some of the line art for the book. Not only did he conceive some of the illustrations, he also modeled some personal protective equipment.

And, finally, thanks to the staff at Brady, especially Danielle Newhouse, whose e-mails reminded me of deadlines and things I needed to complete as soon as possible.

1

In the Beginning
Introduction

OBJECTIVES

At the end of the chapter, the reader will be able to:

1. Describe the effect of the Ryan White CARE Act as it pertains to notifying EMS professionals of an exposure to an infectious agent.
2. Understand the mission statement of the Centers for Disease Control and Prevention (CDC).
3. Understand the mission statement of the Occupational Safety and Health Administration (OSHA).
4. List the general components of OSHA's Bloodborne Pathogens Standard.
5. List the general components of the CDC's Tuberculosis Control Program.
6. Define the term *infectious disease.*
7. List the six links in the chain of infection.
8. List the three infectious agents.
9. List the nine signs or symptoms of an infectious person.

As an EMT or paramedic, every time you respond to a call for help, you put yourself at risk of injury. More recently, that concern has shifted to include the risk for contracting a severe, debilitating, or life-threatening illness. In the early 1980s, the hazards of infectious disease transmission were recognized and the implementation of universal precautions to prevent exposure to bloodborne diseases was begun. Over the years, rules and regulations have been adopted to provide protection from microorganisms that could compromise health. Federal and state regulatory agencies have mandated training in bloodborne pathogens as well as tuberculosis control and prevention. But there are many more diseases "out there" that can cause infection.

WORDS TO KNOW

Bacteria   Single-celled organisms capable of causing an infection.

Exposure   Being subject to or in contact with something such as an infectious agent.

Fungus   An organism found in the soil, air, and water capable of causing a slow-growing infection which, in most cases, is rarely fatal.

Infectious agent   Organisms such as bacteria, viruses, or fungus that can cause infection.

Jaundice   Yellow discoloration of the skin.

Reservoir   A storage place such as a body cavity where infectious agents can be found. The reservoir can be a source of infection for other people.

Virus   An extremely small organism capable of causing infection by replicating (copying) itself using the body's cell material.

The purpose of this book is to provide information about the myriad of infectious diseases that pose a risk in the field. This information is not limited to bloodborne pathogens nor to tuberculosis. This book initially presents information on how diseases are transmitted. It then focuses on how the immune system works to prevent catching a cold or flu even after exposure to one or more people who are highly contagious.

The book then discusses infectious diseases found in childhood. Although some may be immune to these illnesses, many adults have neither had some diseases nor been vaccinated against them. Thus, they are at risk for contracting these diseases common in children. Unfortunately, childhood diseases are more severe in adults.

Following a discussion about childhood diseases, we turn our attention to the diseases seen in adults. As an EMT you will respond to patients with meningitis, tuberculosis, and other serious conditions. Caring for these patients will create risk for contracting the disease. Separate chapters have been included for discussions on HIV and AIDS as well as hepatitis. Another chapter on infectious diseases includes those found in the food we eat. Food poisoning, although not a substantial concern when in contact with patients, does pose some risk for you at work and at home.

Finally, this book presents the key components in an Infection Control Program. Your agency's Infection Control Program is a vital component in protecting against accidental exposure to blood and airborne pathogens. In addition, should exposure occur, your employer's Infection Control Program also provides information on the steps to be taken during the postexposure period.

Is an Infection Control Program really necessary? Consider it as you would "insurance." It's there when you need it. It will protect not only you but also your family and friends from accidental exposure to something that you brought home from the "office."

THE GOVERNMENT MANDATES

In 1990, the U.S. Congress enacted legislation that has become known as the Ryan White Comprehensive AIDS Resource Emergency (CARE) Act. This law, recently reauthorized in 1996 as Public Law 104-146, requires notification of EMS personnel if they may have been exposed to infectious diseases such as HIV, hepatitis, meningitis, and rubella. Should care be provided for an individual who is later determined to have an infectious disease, the receiving hospital is required to notify everyone involved of the risk of exposure. The act also mandates that the employer designate a liaison within the agency to coordinate and facilitate communications and notification in the event of a potential exposure.

Although the Ryan White CARE Act plays an important role in protecting against exposure to infectious diseases, there are two federal agencies whose role is to oversee the control and prevention of infectious diseases—the Centers for Disease Control and Prevention (CDC) and the Occupational Safety and Health Administration (OSHA). These agencies are given the responsibility to provide protection from accidental exposure to illness and injury through rules, regulations, and standards employees and employers must abide by.

Each agency has its own mission statement. The mission statement for the CDC is:

To promote health and quality of life by preventing and controlling disease, injury, and disability.

The Mission Statement for OSHA is:

The mission of the Occupational Safety and Health Administration is to save lives, prevent injuries, and protect the health of America's workers. To accomplish this, federal and state governments must work in partner-

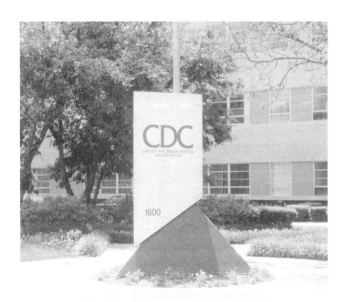

ship with the more than 100 million working men and women and their six and one-half million employers who are covered by the Occupational Safety and Health Act of 1970.

To meet their mission statements, both the CDC and OSHA have developed guidelines or standards that must be used at work. Individual states can mandate similar rules and standards used to provide additional protection from bloodborne pathogens.

Two standards are currently in place that affect EMS employers and their employees. The first is the Bloodborne Pathogens Standard developed by OSHA (29 CFR 1910.1030) that applies to all health-care workers, including EMTs and paramedics. Although this standard is covered in more detail in Chapter 9 on the Infection Control Program, an overview of the Bloodborne Pathogens Standard follows.

Bloodborne Pathogens Standard

Who is covered by the standard. The Standard applies to anyone who is at any risk for exposure to blood or other infectious materials while working. *Exposure* means any subjection to or contact with an infectious material, such as direct contact with the skin, eyes, mucous membranes, or contact through injection.

Exposure control plan. An employer must have an Infection Control Program that identifies who is at risk for exposure, what procedures are in place to reduce the risk of exposure, and a plan to be implemented if an employee is accidentally exposed to a bloodborne pathogen.

Universal precautions, engineering controls, and workplace practice controls. OSHA's Bloodborne Pathogens Standard establishes universal precautions to be used whenever contact occurs with a potentially infectious person. It also identifies ways the employer can reduce the risk of exposure by establishing procedures to handle sharps (needles or bloody instruments). The Standard also calls for policies and procedures to be developed by the employer and used by the employee to reduce risks. For example, employees must always wear disposable latex or vinyl gloves when in contact with a potentially infectious patient.

Personal protective equipment. The Standard requires the employer to issue personal protective equipment that reduces risk of exposure. Disposable gloves, face mask, eye protection, and a gown or protective suit must be immediately available for use. The Standard also calls for a substitute glove for employees who are allergic or sensitive to latex. This equipment is to be issued at no cost to the employee and is to be maintained by the employer.

Training programs. Upon being hired, employees should receive complete training in bloodborne pathogens, OSHA's Standard, and the use of employer-issued personal protective equipment at no cost. Additional training must be provided whenever there is a change in the procedures or a new protective item is issued. Further, this training program must be conducted annually at no cost to the employee.

Vaccinations against hepatitis B. The employer must provide the opportunity to receive the hepatitis B vaccinations at no cost. This series of injections will afford protection from the virus that can cause severe damage to the liver. An employee may choose not to receive the vaccinations. If the employee later changes his or her mind, the employer is responsible for providing the immunizations.

Labeling and handling infectious waste.   The Standard requires the employer to provide appropriate labels, signs, and containers for handling potentially infectious waste such as contaminated laundry and sharps.

Postexposure procedures.   Part of the Infection Control Plan is the procedure to be followed if an employee is exposed to a bloodborne pathogen. The Standard requires a written plan that includes a provision for testing and follow-up care.

Currently, OSHA does not have a Standard for controlling tuberculosis. However, a Standard is being developed and may be implemented over the next few years.
       The CDC has developed guidelines for tuberculosis prevention and control. In 1994, an update to the Tuberculosis Control Program was developed. According to this update, health-care facilities, including EMS agencies, need to adhere to procedures that reduce the risk of exposure to tuberculosis. Highlights of the Tuberculosis Control Program Guidelines follow.

Tuberculosis Control Program Guidelines

Risk assessment.   The employer needs to identify risks for exposure to tuberculosis. The risks can be labeled as *low, medium,* or *high* by assessing the number of tuberculosis patients transported by the EMS agency. Skin testing of those at potential risk for exposure can also help determine the level of risk.

Tuberculosis infection control plan.   The employer needs to have a written plan that identifies all aspects of infection control for tuberculosis. This can be a part of the agency's Infection Control Program.

Respiratory protection.   The employer must provide adequate respiratory protection to be used when in contact with a patient who has tuberculosis. Respiratory protection includes masks meeting CDC criteria for filtering out dust particles that may be contaminated with the bacteria. Masks should fit different face sizes and shapes and should be available in a minimum of three different sizes.

Procedures that may cause the patient to cough.   Suctioning is a procedure that could cause the patient to cough. Do not suction a patient with tuberculosis unless absolutely necessary and only if wearing an appropriate face mask.

Training.   Appropriate training is to be provided in the care and transportation of patients with tuberculosis including the use of personal protective equipment and waste handling. This training is to be offered annually or as needed. Information on airborne pathogens such as tuberculosis can be included in a bloodborne pathogens training program.

Counseling and screening.   If employees are at increased risk for exposure to tuberculosis, the employer should provide them with specific information pertaining to the disease and its signs and symptoms. Periodic skin testing should also be performed if an employee comes in contact with tuberculosis patients.

Evaluation and treatment for infection with tuberculosis.   If an employee is exposed and the skin test reacts positively, the employer needs to provide treatment and follow-up care as needed.

The Employee's Role

The above information has identified many of the responsibilities that the employer must take to protect employees from the hazards of the job. Employees also need to take an active role in making sure they reduce their risk of exposure to an infectious disease. First, they must be aware of the federal, state, and local laws governing infectious diseases and their prevention. Additionally, they need to

- Use universal precautions and the personal protective equipment provided by the employer
- Practice safe techniques in handling hazardous waste such as contaminated needles
- Wash hands after each patient contact

Some of these procedures are inconvenient and others take additional time, causing the EMT to feel that patient care has suffered. But taking the extra minute for personal protection is well worth it, considering the hazards to be faced if the company's Infection Control Program is not followed. Consider . . .

- Was there a time when you did not wear gloves when coming in contact with a patient?
- Was there a time when you did not wear a face mask or eye protection when suctioning a patient's airway or at risk for splashing of body fluids?
- After completing a call and cleaning the equipment, are your hands washed at the hospital or back at the station?
- Do you always wash your hands after using the bathroom?

Infection control programs will work as long as everyone follows the procedures. When a link in the chain breaks, all of the employees, their friends, and their families are at risk for contracting a deadly disease.

INFECTIOUS DISEASES

An *infectious disease* is any disease that can be transmitted from one person to another or from an animal to a person. In order to be considered infectious, several aspects of disease communication must be present. Consider these aspects as links in a chain.

Infectious Agent

For someone to be considered contagious, an organism must be present. A cough containing no viruses or bacteria is not infectious.

Chain of Infection

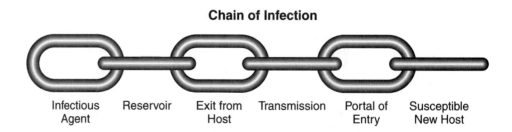

Infectious Agent — Reservoir — Exit from Host — Transmission — Portal of Entry — Susceptible New Host

Reservoir

The infectious person must have a reservoir for the disease. That reservoir can be the sinuses, airways, lungs, or any other body tissues that can harbor the infectious agent.

Portal of Exit

The infectious agent must have a way out of the body. If the organism is in the lungs, coughing can push the disease-causing bacteria or viruses into the air. If the patient's blood is infectious, a cut in the skin allows the organism a way out of the body.

Mode of Transmission

Even if the organism has a way out of the body, it has to have a way of getting to another person. Coughing, sneezing, direct contact with blood or body fluids, or exposure to hazardous waste can bring the organism in contact with someone else.

Portal of Entry

The organism has to have a way to get inside the body. Bacteria on the skin are harmless if they cannot penetrate it. Intact skin is a protective barrier. If the bacteria or virus are on a person's hands and the person rubs his or her eyes, the person has provided the organism a way into the body through the mucous membranes of the eyes. However, washing hands prior to touching sites of entry will help block one of the portals of entry.

Susceptibility

If a person is immune to the organism by vaccination or if the body has a strong resistance to the disease, he or she will not become ill. A person with a strong immune system will fight disease. However, a person whose immune system has been weakened by another disease, by stress, or by other external factors will be more likely to contract the invading disease.

TYPES OF ORGANISMS

There are three main types of infectious agents—bacteria, viruses, and fungi. Each organism has some unique features in its appearance and ways it causes infection.

Bacteria are one-celled organisms that can invade the body and rapidly reproduce causing a severe infection. Bacteria come in three different shapes—rod-shaped bacilli, round sphere cocci, and spiral-shaped spirilla.

Generally speaking, infection by bacteria will depend upon the number of bacteria invading the body and the body's response to them. Bacteria infect first by dividing and multiplying to sufficient numbers. Then they continue to infect by producing enzymes or toxins inside the body that can damage surrounding tissues and impair the body's ability to defend itself. For example, some forms of streptococcus destroy red blood cells by surrounding them or destroying the clots that are attempting to contain or isolate the bacteria.

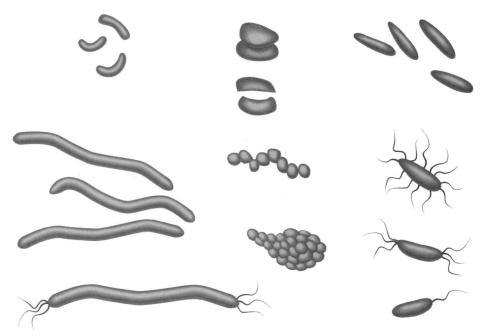

Bacteria come in round, rod, or spiral shapes.

Viruses are extremely small and come in all shapes and sizes. Unlike bacteria, viruses have to make copies or replicas of themselves (replicate). Once inside the body's cell, the virus uses the cell like a factory to make copies of its genetic structure. During this process, the virus can cause the host cell to die. By using the host cell's genetic makeup for its own replication, the virus will ultimately destroy the host cell. This is common with influenza infections.

In another type of viral infection, the genetic structure of the virus becomes incorporated in the host cell's genetics. When the cell reproduces, it reproduces both its own and the virus's genetic structure. In this latent type of infection, new viruses are not immediately produced. Herpes infections are known as latent viral infections.

A third type of viral infection is called the persistent infection. In this type of infection, particles of the virus are shed after the acute stage of the disease has subsided. The host cells are not destroyed. Hepatitis B infection is typical of a persistent infection in which virus particles are being transmitted even though there may be no indication of an acute illness.

When you think about a fungus, you may picture a mushroom, mold, or mildew. Each one is a fungus. As for fungal infections of the body, athlete's foot is a common infection that comes to mind. A fungus is an organism that has cell structures very similar to those of the host.

When encountering a fungus, there are several barriers to prevent it from infecting the body. The natural immunity provided by barriers such as the skin and its fatty acids or mucous membranes and the normal bacteria residing there, makes fungal infection difficult. However, any changes in the skin tissue's natural immunity, such as the use of an antibiotic, may increase the chance of an infection.

Fungi do not produce toxins to cause tissue damage. Rather, they damage the body by directly invading the cells and destroying vital structures. In some cases of severe fungal infection, clumps of fungi can block the airways or, in cases of a fungal infection of the heart, a piece of the fungus structure can dislodge and travel to the brain, causing a stroke.

How can an infectious person be identified? Simply stated, he or she cannot! Some people with latent infections will have no apparent signs and symptoms. Therefore, it is essential that universal precautions be used with every patient.

Other patients however, may give a clue to the risk of exposure by their signs and symptoms. Although not all infectious patients will exhibit any or all of these indications, the index of suspicion should increase when any of the following signs or symptoms are present.

> Fever
> Rash
> Diarrhea
> Vomiting
> Coughing
> Sneezing
> Profuse sweating
> Chills
> Abdominal pain
> Headache with stiff neck
> Jaundice

Fever

A fever is the body's attempt to destroy the infecting organism. Increasing the body's temperature makes the body less hospitable to the invading bacteria or virus.

Rash

Not all rashes indicate an infection. Some rashes may indicate an allergic reaction. However, the presence of a rash should trigger thoughts to enhance infection control, especially if the rash has open sores or draining vesicles.

Diarrhea

Diarrhea does not always mean an infection is present. There are a number of causes of diarrhea. If the diarrhea is accompanied by any other indication of an infection, such as fever, it could indicate a serious gastrointestinal infection.

Vomiting

As with diarrhea, vomiting alone does not indicate the presence of an infectious disease. Consider other possibilities when the patient complains of nausea and vomiting. If the patient also has a fever and other indications of an infection, consider the patient contagious.

Coughing

Coughing, especially when there is tightness or congestion in the chest, can signal the presence of an infection. Respiratory precautions should be used.

Sneezing

A simple sneeze may be a means of eliminating an irritant from the nose or sinuses. If the patient is sneezing due to a cold or flu, respiratory precautions are in order.

Profuse Sweating

A patient who is sweating when there is no obvious reason for it could have a fever and should be considered infectious.

Chills

Chills, often accompanied by shivering at normal room temperature, are an indication of a fever.

Abdominal Pain

Abdominal cramping or pain accompanied by vomiting or diarrhea can signal the presence of a severe gastrointestinal infection. Handle soiled linens and clothing carefully.

Headache with Stiff Neck

The stiff neck should trigger concern for meningitis. Although it is not possible to determine the presence of bacterial or viral meningitis in the field, treat any patient with a headache, stiff neck, and fever as a significant risk for infection.

Jaundice

Jaundice, or the yellow discoloration of the skin, is a sign of a problem with the liver, gallbladder, or blood. Be alert for exposure to hepatitis.

Universal precautions make the assumption that every patient is at risk for infection. By using personal protective equipment when coming in contact with patients showing signs and symptoms of infectious disease, risk of exposure will be reduced.

☎ YOU MAKE THE CALL

You have responded to a call for help where you found a 29-year-old man huddled over the toilet bowl vomiting. When you ask him about his condition, he looks up and in a very slurred speech says, "I don't feel good." You determine from friends and family that the man had recently become intoxicated while watching a football game on television. This is somewhat confirmed by the odor of an alcoholic beverage in the man's vomit.

Is this man's vomiting indicative of an infectious disease?

Because he doesn't show any outward signs of an infectious disease, would it be permissible not to wear gloves while examining or treating this patient?

SUMMARY

This chapter introduced you to the world of communicable diseases and infection control. At the start of the chapter, you were told about what information this book will provide you about infectious diseases and reducing your risk for exposure.

The chapter presented the governmental mandates that help ensure a safe working environment. In the business of prehospital care, there is no risk-free workplace. Every call presents inherent dangers. OSHA and the CDC have developed Standards and guidelines to help make the job a bit safer. These were highlighted to give a better understanding of the regulations that employers and employees must meet.

The chapter also discussed the definition of an infectious disease and the links in the chain leading to infection. The host must have an infectious agent that has a way out of his or her body and a way into another. In addition, the person has to be susceptible to that infectious agent.

The nature of infectious organisms was briefly discussed. The three main organisms include bacteria, viruses, and fungi—each with its own way of infecting an individual.

Finally, some general signs and symptoms of an infectious person were listed and discussed. Always assume that every patient poses a risk and always apply the principles of universal precautions.

Let's be very careful out there!

2

Going My Way?
Modes of Disease Transmission

OBJECTIVES

At the end of the chapter, the reader will be able to:

1. Define the following terms:

   Airborne infection   Droplet infection

   Exposure   Infectious

   Transmission   Vector-borne infection

2. Given a list of modes of transmission, correctly indicate that coughing is a means of transmitting a disease by indirect contact.

3. Given a list of modes of transmission, correctly indicate that kissing is a means of transmitting a disease by direct contact.

4. Describe how wearing gloves can protect against infectious disease transmission.

5. Describe how wearing a face mask can protect against infectious disease transmission.

6. Describe how wearing goggles can protect against infectious disease transmission.

7. Describe how wearing a gown or protective suit can protect against infectious disease transmission.

In order to become exposed to or infected by a communicable disease, the virus, bacteria, or fungus has to have a way of transferring from the contagious person to someone else. This is what is meant by *mode of transmission*—how the disease is transmitted from the person who is ill. This chapter presents information about factors affecting disease transmission and the various modes of transmission that typically allow an infectious agent a way of traveling from one person to another.

WORDS TO KNOW

Airborne infection   Infection caused by inhaling viruses or bacteria carried in the air.

Contagious   Characteristic of a disease that is able to be transferred from one person or source to another person.

Droplet infection   Infection by inhaling droplets of moisture carrying bacteria or viruses.

Dustborne infection   Infection by inhaling particles of dust to which bacteria or viruses are attached.

Exposure   A condition that allows a person to be subjected to an infectious disease. An exposure does not mean an infection has occurred.

Infectious   Characteristic of a microorganism's ability to cause an infection by invading the body and multiplying in the body's tissues.

Portal of entry   A location where the infectious agent can invade the body. A portal of entry can be an open wound, the eyes, the airways, the gastrointestinal tract, or other organ system.

Susceptible   Characteristic of a person lacking the ability to fight or resist the invading virus or bacteria.

Transmission   The passing of a disease from one person or source to another person.

Vector-borne infection   The transfer of an infectious agent from one person or source to another by a carrier such as an insect.

KEY CONCEPTS

In order to better understand the concept of disease transmission, we need to have a grasp on some key concepts of infectious diseases. Disease transmission means the transfer of a disease from one individual to another or from an animal or other source to a person. But, in order to be at risk, several criteria must be met.

First, the disease must be contagious, meaning it must be capable of being spread from someone else or another source. Basically, the disease must have a way out of the host.

Second, it must have a means of transportation or mode of transmission so that it can move from one site to another.

Third, it must have a way into the body. The bacteria or virus must have a portal of entry such as an open wound, path into the respiratory system, or other avenue such as the gastrointestinal system.

Fourth, the disease must also be considered infectious or capable of invading the body and causing damage to the tissues or cells. If an agent such as a bacteria or virus comes in contact with the body, it must have a sufficient number of "bugs" to cause infection. If only a few viruses come in contact with the skin, the chances of their ability to infect are minimal.

Fifth, the individual must be susceptible to the invading organism. If the immune system is working optimally or there is an acquired immunity to the organism, the chance of infection is reduced. If, however, health is poor or the immune system is compromised, the bacteria or virus could more easily cause infection.

Finally, there is a difference between being exposed to a disease and being infected by it. Just because a person has been exposed to a disease does not mean that he or she has been infected. Remember, a disease is infectious or a person is infected only if the organism can invade the body and multiply. Several barriers to the disease's entry render the organism inactive. See Chapter 3 for information on the immune system as well as barriers against invading organisms.

There are several ways an infectious agent can be transferred from one person to another. The modes of transmission include airborne transmission, direct contact, indirect contact, and vector-borne.

Airborne Transmission

One of the more common methods of transmission is airborne infection. In cases of airborne infection, the person inhales bacteria or viruses that have been suspended in air, on water droplets, or on dust particles.

Organisms can be transmitted to a person if they are carried by currents of air. In many cases, the organisms are attached to a droplet of moisture or a particle of dust, but this is not always necessary. We consider droplet infection the most common form of communicating infectious agents between people. In a droplet infection, moisture from the respiratory system containing infectious material is expelled into the air when the infected person coughs or sneezes. A person with an upper respiratory infection has a reservoir of infectious material in the airways and lungs. When he or she sneezes, bacterial or virus-laden moisture from the airways is expelled into the air (see photograph below). The force of air from the cough or sneeze, or the currents of air transfer the infectious agent to others in the immediate area.

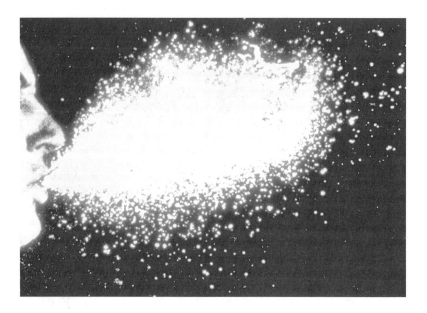

Infectious agents can attach themselves to particles of dust that are distributed in an area whenever the air is disturbed by the wind or a person passing nearby. The dust particles are transferred to the other person when they are inhaled or when they contact broken skin.

Direct Contact

Another means by which an infectious agent can be transmitted from one person to another is through direct contact—straight from person to person. An example of direct contact includes kissing where there is contact with the infected person's mucous membranes. Sexual relations is another form of direct contact. Direct contact occurs when there is a pathway between the infected person's reservoir and the other person's portal of entry.

Direct contact can also occur during exposure to a patient's blood or feces. A patient's blood dripping onto an open wound or splashing into the eyes are examples of direct contact. Fecal-oral contact is a well-known mode of transmitting hepatitis. By touching a patient's feces, either on the patient's body or on soiled linens, you can become exposed and possibly risk infection. If the hands are contaminated with feces, smoking or eating can put the fecal matter into the mouth where it can begin its invasion of the body. Therefore, it is important to wash the hands thoroughly after contact with any patient.

Indirect Contact

Direct contact with an infected person is not the only way to bring bacteria or viruses into the body. Another method of exposure to an infectious agent is known as indirect contact. By touching surfaces that have been contaminated with the bacteria or virus, infection can spread. Using food utensils or cups or glasses that were used by an infectious person can introduce the agent into the body.

Some contaminated surfaces that might harbor bacteria or viruses include telephone receivers, door handles, paper towel dispensers, faucets, sink drains, and kitchen cutting boards. One surface that we rarely consider as a source for indirect contact is the steering wheel of the emergency vehicle. Consider the last patient who may have had a communicable disease. Following approved department practices, the EMTs were wearing gloves while in contact with the patient. After caring for the patient and placing him or her onto the gurney, they loaded the gurney into the ambulance for transportation. Were the gloves removed before the EMT climbed into the driver's seat and headed to the emergency department? If not, contaminants were left on the steering wheel that would be transferred to the driver's bare hands after the call—when the patient and his or her condition have been forgotten.

In addition to contact with a contaminated surface, indirect contact can also be in the form of waterborne infection. Swimming in water contaminated by a sewage spill is inviting disaster. Hepatitis A has been known to be transmitted by shellfish that have been living in sewage-contaminated water.

Vector-Borne Transmission

Infectious agents can also be transmitted from one host or source to another by a "common carrier." Animal and insect bites can transmit a variety of diseases from infected animals to a person. Rabies, Lyme disease, Rocky Mountain spotted fever, and malaria are just a few examples of vector-borne diseases.

Animal bites are not the only means of vector-borne infections. Blood transfusions, receiving blood products or organs, and needle-stick injuries can also pose a risk of infection.

☎ **YOU MAKE THE CALL**

You respond to a retirement community where you see an 80-year-old man sitting on the edge of his bed seeming to have trouble breathing. He is coughing and between the coughs you hear congestion in his chest. Occasionally, the man coughs up sputum, which he spits into a tissue. He tosses the tissue into the wastebasket next to his bed. The man tells you he has a fever and aches "all over." He also tells you that many of the people in the community have had the flu.

In this situation, list the ways the influenza virus can be transmitted.
What personal protective equipment can be used to reduce risk of exposure?
Will a flu shot completely prevent contracting the disease?

PROTECTING AGAINST INFECTION

There are several means by which EMS professionals can protect themselves to prevent disease from being transmitted. The first is through the use of protective personal equipment such as gloves, masks, goggles, and gowns or suits. Using these items will prevent the transmission of a disease. Chapter 9, Putting It All Together, discusses these items in more detail.

Gloves reduce the risk of direct and indirect transmission of the bacteria or viruses by placing a barrier between the skin and the infectious agent.

A face mask will reduce the risk of transferring the disease via airborne transmission. For most infectious diseases, a simple surgical face mask will suffice. However, when in contact with patients with tuberculosis, a specially designed face mask will filter out the smallest water droplets and dust particles that could be contaminated with microorganisms. Specialty equipment will be discussed later in this book.

Using goggles reduces the risk of direct contact with bloodborne pathogens. Wearing goggles prevents blood or other body fluids from being splashed into the eyes, blocking the portal of entry into the body.

Finally, a gown or protective suit will also act as a barrier against the transmission of infectious agents, especially if there is substantial risk of contact with blood or other body fluids with clothing.

Using personal protective equipment and following the guidelines mandating its use under specific circumstances will reduce risk of exposure to a potentially life-threatening blood or airborne pathogen.

SUMMARY

Bacteria, viruses, and fungi can be transmitted from one person to another or from an animal to a person by any number of methods. In order for the transfer to be successful, several key components must be in place. These key aspects include the presence of a contagious disease; a viable method of transferring the disease; a portal of entry or way into the body; the ability to invade the body and cause cell or tissue damage; and host susceptibility. If any of these essential aspects are missing, a disease cannot be successfully transmitted to another person.

There are various ways a contagious disease can be transmitted from one person to another. These include airborne transmission of the agent either alone or attached to water or dust, direct contact, indirect contact, and vector transmission. Interfering with any means of transferring the infectious agent— using personal protective equipment—will prevent the disease from being transmitted to another person.

Catch as Catch Can't!

The Immune System

OBJECTIVES

At the end of the chapter, the reader will be able to:

1. Define the following terms:

Antibody	Antigen
Leukocyte	Lymphocyte
Macrophage	Neutrophil
T-cytotoxic lymphocytes	T-helper lymphocytes

2. Describe the role of the mouth in protecting against infection.
3. Describe the role of the gastrointestinal system in protecting against infection.
4. Describe the role of the respiratory system in protecting against infection.
5. Describe how the skin protects the body against invading bacteria.
6. Describe the inflammatory response the body has after bacteria have been able to invade the body through the skin.
7. Describe the role of neutrophils and macrophages during the inflammatory response.
8. State how a person develops an acquired immunity.
9. Describe the role of B-lymphocytes in protecting the body against an infectious agent.
10. Describe the role of T-lymphocytes in protecting the body against an infectious agent.
11. List three steps that can be taken to assist the immune system in protecting against disease.
12. Discuss the role of immunization in protecting against illnesses.

A person coughs. Another person sneezes. Someone has just been exposed to the worst cold virus ever and assumes that he or she will be coughing, hacking, wheezing, and sneezing soon. Several days pass and the exposure is forgotten because there has been no hint of the sniffles or any indication of a developing upper respiratory infection. The body has successfully defended itself against an army of invading bacteria or viruses.

In order for an infection to develop, the attacking organism must have a way of getting into the body and, once there, must have the ability to overcome the body's defenses. The body uses three mechanisms to prevent or resist an infection—natural barriers, an inflammatory response, and the immune system. The purpose of this chapter is to overview the natural defenses the body uses to protect itself from the multitude of viruses, bacteria, and fungi that

WORDS TO KNOW

Agglutination   The clumping together of cells.

Antibody   A specific molecule that has the ability to adhere to and interact only with the antigen that stimulates the antibody's production.

Antigen   A substance capable of inducing an immune response. Antigens include bacteria, viruses, and tissue cells.

B-lymphocytes   A type of white blood cell (leukocyte) specifically responsible for the production and secretion of antibodies.

Cilia   Hairlike structures extending from a cell that beat rhythmically to move fluid or mucus over the cell.

Leukocytes   White blood cells that act as scavengers and help fight infections.

Lymphocyte   A member of the white blood cells that make up the body's immune system and the precursors of the immune system. Lymphocytes are primarily located in the lymph nodes and lymph-like tissues throughout the body.

Lysis   The destruction of a cell.

Macrophages   Originating in the bone marrow, these cells, when activated at the site of an infection, attack and ingest foreign cells including bacteria and viruses.

Neutrophil   A white blood cell that can attack and destroy bacteria or viruses circulating in the blood.

Phagocytosis   The process of engulfing and ingesting foreign particles such as bacteria or viruses.

T-cytotoxic lymphocytes   Killer cells—lymphocytes responsible for killing cells bearing a specific kind of antigen.

T-helper lymphocytes   Lymphocytes that help recognize certain antigens and stimulate the production of T-cytotoxic lymphocytes.

T-suppressor lymphocytes   Lymphocytes that suppress antibody production as well as the production and function of T-helper and T-cytotoxic lymphocytes.

Vasodilation   Opening or widening of blood vessels to allow the passage of more blood.

threaten us daily. These defenses include our natural barriers, the body's inflammatory response, and the immune system. It also presents information on how to remain more resistant to the microorganisms around us.

NATURAL BARRIERS

The first line of defense consists of natural barriers. The skin presents a great barrier to organisms that are trying to enter the body. However, there are other barriers in the respiratory and gastrointestinal systems that fight potential infection. See the following illustration on natural barriers.

The skin, when intact, presents a tremendous blockade against bacteria, viruses, and fungi. Moisture and oils from sweat and sebaceous glands contain organic or fatty acids that inhibit bacterial growth. The outermost layer of skin, the epidermis, is continually shedding and being replaced by new layers. As layers of epidermis are lost, they take the infectious agents with them.

In the respiratory system, airflow and the mucous membranes act as natural barriers. When exposed to droplet infection, the inhaled droplets are initially trapped in the mucus that lines the upper airways. In the nasal passages, mucus provides a chemical and physical barrier to viruses and bacteria. When the organisms are trapped in the mucus, they can be removed from the body by a sneeze. In the lower respiratory system, a cough might be an initial means of defense. Invading foreign substances can trigger a cough reflex, expelling mucus and infectious fluids from the airways. Mucus as well as the mechanical

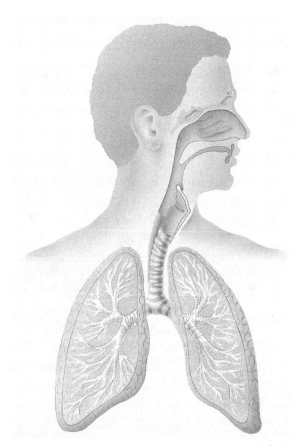

The respiratory system provides protection against infectious organisms through its natural barriers.

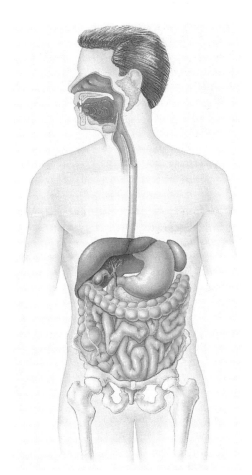

The gastrointestinal system offers natural barriers against invading bacteria and viruses.

action of the cilia that line the airways helps trap and remove organisms. Cilia move the mucus up toward the mouth where it can be coughed up and either swallowed or expelled, protecting the airways and lungs from infection.

In the gastrointestinal system, the salivary glands produce fluid and enzymes that, in combination with movement of the tongue, can flush and destroy several types of infectious agents. The stomach, with its hydrochloric acid and low pH, can also kill microorganisms. In the small bowel, bile acids, and in the lower gastrointestinal tract, fatty acids, serve as chemical barriers to infection. Finally, peristalsis of the bowel and the flow of liquids through the intestines can assist in ridding the gut of unwanted bacteria and viruses.

Each of the above organ systems provides defenses against infection. However, these barriers might not be working at full capacity or may have been affected by injury or another disease process. For example, if the skin has been injured by trauma, such as a burn or cut, bacteria encounter less resistance and can enter the body more readily. When this happens, a second barrier or level of resistance is used—the inflammatory response.

INFLAMMATORY RESPONSE

If the invading microorganisms have survived the body's initial defenses and penetrated underlying tissues, the body can invoke the inflammatory response. The body has the unique ability to identify and destroy infectious agents using

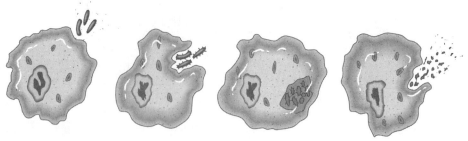

Phagocytosis

its white blood cells (leukocytes). Certain white blood cells (neutrophils and macrophages) attack and ingest the invading agent in a process known as *phagocytosis.*

A typical inflammatory response of the skin has a distinctive appearance—hot, swollen, and red. Similar to the response on the skin, an inflammatory response can occur in deeper tissues. An inflammatory response is characterized initially by vasodilation in the area of the invasion. With increased blood flow to the specific area, capillaries become engorged and tend to leak fluid, allowing the fluid and cells to accumulate. Chemical substances in the injured tissues attract neutrophils and macrophages, which will attack and devour the invading agent within minutes. This devouring of infectious agents occurs everywhere in the body including the skin, lymph nodes, lungs, liver, spleen, and bone marrow. If the infection is more severe, the body will respond with an increase in the number of neutrophils and macrophages sent to the area.

As the neutrophils and macrophages accumulate, attack, and destroy the infectious agents and dead or injured tissues, they will eventually die. The dead neutrophils and macrophages along with tissue fluids will collect in the area of the infection. This liquid accumulation is known as *pus.* After the infection has been stopped, the pus will gradually be absorbed into the surrounding tissues and leave only a residual evidence of the infection.

One of the results of the inflammatory process is to close or wall off the injured area and separate it from the rest of the tissues. The purpose of walling off the infection is to delay or prevent the spread of the infectious agent to the rest of the body.

THE IMMUNE SYSTEM

Although all of the defense mechanisms mentioned earlier are actually components of the body's immune system, we often think of the immune system in terms of what is referred to as acquired immunity—a specific resistance against particular invading infectious agents. Briefly stated, acquired immunity is a special component of the body's lymphocyte system that creates antibodies and activates specialized lymphocytes to fight a given bacteria or virus.

Lymphocytes are primarily located in the lymph nodes and lymph-like tissues (spleen, gastrointestinal tract, and bone marrow). These tissues are strategically and advantageously located throughout the body to intercept invading microorganisms before they can spread.

There are two categories of acquired immunity. Both types are closely aligned, but each works in its own separate way. The first type consists of cells called B-lymphocytes that produce antibodies. When activated, these antibodies attack and destroy the invading organism. The second type of immunity is referred to as the T-cell or T-lymphocyte immunity. When an invading organism is recognized by the body, this system activates large quantities of lymphocytes that are designed to identify and destroy the organism.

In order for acquired immunity to develop, the body must be exposed to the infectious agent either by infection or by vaccination. Without such exposure, the body will not be able to recognize the organism as foreign and the organism will, if not stopped by phagocytosis, be allowed to continue the infection.

Antibodies

When an infectious agent enters the body, it is called an *antigen*—a substance that begins the process of acquired immunity. During the initial or first exposure to the antigen, the immune system creates substances known as antibodies. These substances are designed to specifically recognize the antigen should it invade the body in the future. If the toxin, bacteria, or virus attempts to enter the body again, the antibodies are immediately activated and respond in two different ways. The first is by directly attacking and destroying the antigen. A second response involves a complex mechanism of actions known as a *complement system*. The antibodies and its complement system can destroy or inactivate the organism in several different ways including:

- *Phagocytosis.* Stimulating the neutrophils and macrophages to surround and ingest the organism.
- *Lysis or destruction.* Rupturing the organism's cell wall and destroying the cell.
- *Agglutination or clumping.* Causing the invading organisms to stick to each other and form clumps of organisms making them unable to continue infecting the body.
- *Neutralizing.* The immune system attacks the structures of the virus cells and neutralizes them. Once neutralized, they are not able to infect.
- *Inflammatory response.* The inflammatory response that has been described above causes macrophages and neutrophils to appear and ingest the antigens.

T-Lymphocytes

Along with the antibodies, the immune system has a second type of acquired immunity—through specifically designed and activated lymphocytes that destroy the microorganism. This part of the immune system is referred to as the *T-lymphocyte system.* There are three different types of T cells: T-helper cells, T-cytotoxic cells, and T-suppressor cells, each playing a key role in stimulating the immune system to destroy an invading agent.

T-helper cells. T-helper cells are the most numerous of the T-lymphocytes. Their primary function is to help the immune system as regulators of the immune system's functions. To accomplish their job, T-helper cells form different proteins that affect other cells in the immune system. You may have heard of these proteins that have been called interleukins and interferons. These proteins stimulate the production of the two other T-lymphocytes—T-cytotoxic and T-suppressor cells.

Another effect of T-helper cells is to assist in the formation of antibodies. Without T-helper cells, the creation of antibodies is significantly impaired. Again, an infection can spread through the body with minimal resistance.

When the T-helper cells have been destroyed or inactivated, the immune system is virtually paralyzed. In HIV infections, T-helper cells are destroyed, allowing the spread of opportunistic infections in the AIDS patient. For example, when the T-helper cells are inactivated or destroyed, they cannot produce the proteins responsible for producing other T-cells.

T-cytotoxic cells. T-cytotoxic cells are also known as T-killer cells. The T-killer cells bind with the cell of the invading organism and drill a hole into the cell wall. The organism's cell fluid leaks from this hole and destroys it. Further, the T-killer cells release substances and digestive enzymes into the organism. These substances, known as cytotoxic (killer) substances, cause the attacked cell to swell and, ultimately, dissolve. A nice feature is that T-cytotoxic cells are not limited in the number of invading cells they can attack. After binding with, punching holes in, and delivering enzymes to one victim cell, they can release and move on to another victim.

T-suppressor cells. Another type of T-lymphocyte is called the T-suppressor cell. The T-suppressor cell is responsible for limiting the actions of both T-helper and T-cytotoxic cells, preventing them from damaging the normal parts of the body. It is important for the immune system to be able to recognize normal body cells and destroy the unusual or nonbody (foreign or invading) cells without affecting healthy tissues. Unfortunately, there are times when the T-suppressor cells do not function properly or adequately and the body develops an immunity to itself, resulting in what is called an autoimmune disease. Autoimmune diseases include rheumatic fever, glomerulonephritis, myasthenia gravis, multiple sclerosis, insulin-dependent diabetes mellitus, and lupus erythematosus.

HELPING THE IMMUNE SYSTEM

How can the immune system be helped and reduce the chances of infection? As will be discussed later in this book, using universal precautions and washing hands after contact with any patient will reduce the possibility of infection. However, patient contact is not the only source of potential contamination. There are risks from things we do not suspect.

To reduce the chances of infection from contact with a potential source of contamination, the skin must be protected. Washing hands is important after any contact with a potentially infected surface or substance. If the hands have small cuts and scrapes, protect those areas by cleaning them, applying an antimicrobial ointment, and covering with a dressing as needed. This is also true for other areas of the body that could be at risk from small cuts or nicks from shaving. If hands are dry and tend to become chafed, moisturize the skin with any one of several lotions. If in doubt as to what lotion to use, contact a physician or dermatologist for advice.

To enhance internal barriers and the immune system, several methods will increase protection. These include eating properly, getting sufficient rest, decreasing stress, and getting immunized against common infectious agents.

Eat properly. Good nutrition is essential in helping the body defend against invading microorganisms. The body needs proper nutrition to develop blood cells, promote bone growth, and enhance the immune system. For help with a diet or to obtain information about using supplemental vitamins, contact a doctor or seek nutritional counseling.

Get plenty of rest and reduce stress. Lack of rest and unabated stress can weaken the immune system, leading to both minor and major diseases. A person under a lot of stress finds he or she is continuously fighting off repeated colds. A physician or counselor can help identify effective ways of coping with and reducing the stress.

Get vaccinated. Vaccinations have been developed for many diseases, including most of the childhood diseases. Immunizations have been developed for smallpox, polio, measles, mumps, rubella, chickenpox, hepatitis B, and others. Contact a physician and ask about the immunizations. Health-care workers are strongly urged to consider an annual flu shot given to reduce chances of contracting influenza.

SUMMARY

This chapter has given an overview of the body's defense systems that help it fight infection. The defenses used to ward off invading microorganisms include our natural barriers such as the skin and the lining of the respiratory and gastrointestinal systems.

Should an infectious agent penetrate these barriers, a second line of defense can prevent their taking over. This second line of defense is an inflammatory process in that physical and chemical reactions allow the body's leukocytes to attack and destroy the bacteria or viruses.

Finally, the body uses its acquired immunity to defend itself. The B- and T-lymphocyte systems produce antibodies as well as specialized T-lymphocytes to attack and destroy invading bacteria or viruses.

The immune system needs help to maintain its functions. Exhaustion, poor diet, and unabated stress can inhibit this valuable protective system. With adequate rest and nutrition along with stress reduction and immunizations, the body's defenses can be strengthened, reducing the risk of infection.

4

Out of the Mouths of Babes
Communicable Diseases of Childhood

OBJECTIVES

At the end of the chapter, the reader will be able to:

1. Define the following terms:

Conjunctivitis	Dysphagia
Dyspnea	Hypoxia
Inspiratory stridor	Koplik's spots
Laryngotracheobronchiolitis	Macule
Otitis media	Papule

2. State the mode of transmission of each of the following diseases:

Varicella	Croup
Diphtheria	Impetigo
Respiratory syncytial virus	Mumps
Rubella	Rubeola

3. List the signs, symptoms, and complications of chickenpox.
4. List the signs and symptoms of German measles.
5. State why German measles is a serious condition when contracted during the first three months of pregnancy.
6. List the signs and symptoms of the measles.
7. List the signs, symptoms, and complications of the mumps.
8. List the signs or symptoms of croup.
9. List the signs or symptoms of epiglottitis.
10. List the signs or symptoms of respiratory syncytial virus.
11. Describe the three stages and sound of whooping cough.
12. Describe the condition known as paralytic polio.
13. List three signs or symptoms of diphtheria.
14. State the mode of transmission and appearance of conjunctivitis.
15. Describe the appearance of impetigo.

Many of us have been exposed to the myriad of communicable diseases of childhood. A disease is contracted and then, after it has run its course, forgotten. Many receive vaccinations and never contract the disease.

Childhood diseases are numerous and, once they have run their course, the body develops a lifelong immunity to the disease. This immunity is from the creation of antibodies that recognize future exposures and destroy the viruses or bacteria before they can actually cause infection. Another form of protection against childhood diseases is through immunization. The Advisory Committee on Immunization Practices (ACIP), the American Academy of Pediatrics (AAP), and the American Academy of Family Physicians (AAFP) have developed and approved a childhood immunization schedule to protect against common infectious diseases. More information will be presented later in this chapter.

WORDS TO KNOW

Cyanosis   A bluish discoloration of the skin that indicates low oxygen levels in the blood.

Conjunctivitis   Inflammation of the lining of the eyelids.

Dysphagia   Difficulty or painful swallowing.

Diphtheria   A highly contagious bacterial disease that affects the membranes of the throat and, if not treated, can affect other organs of the body.

Dyspnea   The sensation of difficult or labored breathing.

Encephalopathy   A degenerative disease of the brain.

H. influenzae   A bacterial agent often responsible for epiglottitis.

Hepatitis   Inflammation of the liver.

Hypoxia   Abnormally low oxygen level in the arterial blood.

Inspiratory stridor   Crowing sound heard when a patient with narrowed upper airways inhales.

Koplik's spots   Small, irregular bright red spots with a bluish-white speck in the center of the spot found in the mouth of patients with measles.

Laryngotracheobronchiolitis   Inflammation of the larynx, trachea, bronchi, and bronchioles. Also known as croup.

Macule   A discolored spot on the skin that is not raised or elevated.

Mastitis   Inflammation of the breast.

Meninges   The layers of tissue covering the brain and spinal cord.

Myocarditis   Inflammation of the heart muscle.

Nephritis   Inflammation of the kidney.

Otitis media   Inflammation of the middle ear, common in childhood, that has a variety of causes.

Pancreatitis   Inflammation of the pancreas.

Papule   A small, rounded elevation in the skin.

Parainfluenza virus   A virus that has been found in the airways of patients with upper respiratory infection.

Parotitis   Inflammation of the parotid salivary gland. These glands are the largest of the salivary glands and are located on either side of the face, in front of and below the ears.

Paroxysms Sudden recurrences or spasms. A paroxysm of coughing is repeated coughing from 5 to 15 coughs.

Pericardium The sac surrounding the heart.

Pertussis Whooping cough.

Poliomyelitis A viral disease that can result in residual weakness or paralysis.

Prostatitis Inflammation of the prostate gland.

Pseudomembrane A false membrane. It appears as a layer of tissue but does not have the same characteristics.

Pustule A small, elevated lesion of the skin that contains pus.

Respiratory syncytial virus A major cause of upper respiratory infections of children.

Rhinitis Inflammation of the lining of the nose and nasal passageways that can lead to a runny nose or nasal stuffiness.

Rotavirus A virus which causes diarrhea in infants and children.

Rubella German measles.

Rubeola Measles.

Trimester A three-month period of time during a pregnancy.

Tripod position A position in which there is a three-point support using the buttocks and hands as the three points. The result is to elevate the shoulders to make breathing easier.

Varicella Another name for chickenpox, a viral disease causing a rash.

Vesicles A small elevation of the skin containing fluid.

EMS professionals will come in contact with children with childhood diseases. For most, this poses no problem. However, for those who may never have had a particular disease, contracting it as an adult can pose serious or even critical health problems. The purpose of this chapter is to discuss childhood diseases, their cause, method of transmission, and general signs and symptoms. The chapter will also offer suggestions for EMS personnel to protect themselves in cases where they are at risk for contracting an illness.

CHICKENPOX (VARICELLA)

Nature and Spread of the Disease

Chickenpox, formally known as varicella, is more frequently seen in winter and spring. It is caused by a virus generally spread by droplet infection as well as direct contact. A child playing in the home of an infected and contagious child can be easily exposed to the virus. A child can be considered contagious for approximately two weeks, generally starting about two days prior to the rash appearing, ending when all the vesicles have scabbed over.

Signs and Symptoms

Children with chickenpox complain of a mild headache, decreased appetite, and have a moderate fever that can develop from 11 to 15 days after exposure. Approximately 24 hours later, the rash of chickenpox appears. The rash in most cases of chickenpox involves the trunk; however, in severe cases, the face and internal structures can be affected.

Initially, the rash looks like a reddish, flat discoloration on the skin. Within a few hours, the rash progresses to itchy vesicles containing clear fluid that are raised above a reddened base. These vesicles have been described as looking like a "dew drop on a rose petal." In about six to eight hours, the vesicles begin to crust. As some vesicles crust, new crops of lesions may begin to appear. The acute phase of the disease will last from four to seven days. New vesicles stop appearing around day five and in three weeks the disease has run its course.

Children tolerate chickenpox rather well and rarely develop a severe case of the disease or any complications associated with the infection. But adults, especially those whose immune systems are compromised, can experience a severe and potentially fatal case of varicella. Vesicles can appear in the mouth, throat, upper airways, eyelids, rectum, and vagina. Vesicles in the mouth and throat can cause dysphagia (difficult or painful swallowing) whereas vesicles in the airways may cause severe dyspnea, requiring advanced airway support.

Complications associated with chickenpox include secondary infections of the ruptured vesicles by streptococcus or staphylococcus bacteria. Pneumonia is a common complication of chickenpox in adults, newborn children, and patients with compromised immune systems. Other complications, although rare, include myocarditis, hepatitis, and encephalopathy.

Personal Protection

One of the biggest protective mechanisms is having the disease as a child. As was mentioned above, contracting the disease in childhood offers lifelong immunity in the event of future exposures. A person who has not had chickenpox as a child can be vaccinated against the disease.

On the scene when caring for a child with chickenpox, using universal precautions such as gloves is recommended. Be careful with the vesicles because rupturing them can spread the infection. Applying cool, wet compresses to itching skin may decrease the child's tendency to scratch and rupture the vesicles. Those who have not developed an immunity or been vaccinated should use a face mask to provide protection from droplet infection. As always, a thorough washing of hands is required after patient care has been completed.

GERMAN MEASLES (RUBELLA)

Nature and Spread of the Disease

German measles, more formally known as rubella (also known as three-day measles), is a common childhood viral illness typically prevalent in the spring. Like chickenpox, having the disease usually provides a lifelong immunity to German measles. It should be noted, however, that occasional subsequent rubella infections have been reported in people who have either had the illness or have been vaccinated against it. The disease is transmitted by droplet infection. A person with German measles is considered contagious for a week prior to the appearance of the rash and ending a week after the rash disappears.

Signs and Symptoms

After a two- to three-week incubation period, the onset of the illness begins with a short period of fatigue and general uneasiness. Shortly thereafter, a rash appears on the face and neck and spreads quickly to the trunk. The rash consists of a reddened spot with a small raised area. The rash is accompanied by a flushed appearance of the skin. Lymph nodes in the neck may be swollen and tender in younger children. The rash fades within three days.

Other signs and symptoms are very mild and may be overlooked. These signs and symptoms, particularly in the adult with German measles, include fever, headache, joint pain or stiffness, and a mild case of rhinitis or irritation of the nasal passages with stuffiness and perhaps a runny nose.

Complications of German measles are rare; however, the disease poses a significant threat to women who are pregnant. A woman in the early stages of pregnancy who contracts rubella is at significant risk for spontaneous abortion or stillbirth. Significant birth defects have been reported in children born of mothers having the disease in the first trimester (three months) of pregnancy.

Personal Protection

Personal protection should consist of universal precautions and washing your hands after patient care. Additional precautions should be undertaken by EMS professionals who may be pregnant. A vaccination is available to prevent German measles and is recommended for women of childbearing age.

MEASLES (RUBEOLA)

Nature and Spread of the Disease

Measles, also known as rubeola, is a very contagious viral disease spread by droplet infection as well as direct contact. The disease can be transmitted to others from two to four days prior to the appearance of the rash. Like chickenpox, once you have had measles, you have a lifelong immunity. This is not the case after immunization with the measles vaccine. Outbreaks of the disease have been reported in previously immunized people.

Signs and Symptoms

The illness consists of two stages. The first stage appears after an incubation period of approximately one to two weeks. The patient will have a fever, runny nose, cough, and conjunctivitis (inflammation of the lining of the eyelids). The fever tends to increase slightly each day. The patient may also complain of headache and neck pain.

Two to four days after the onset of the measles, the second stage begins—characterized by spots appearing in the patient's mouth. Koplik's spots, as they are called, look like small grains of salt or white sand surrounded by a reddened area. Inflammation of the throat, larynx, and trachea can develop.

One to two days after Koplik's spots appear, the patient develops the rash characteristic of the measles. The rash begins in front of and below the ears, quickly spreading to the neck, face, trunk, arms, and legs. The rash appears to be a small reddened area that, as it progresses, develops a small papule or raised area. Itching associated with the rash is generally mild. The fever continues and, at the height of the illness, may approach 104 degrees.

Swelling around the eyes may occur along with conjunctivitis, and the patient may be sensitive to light, preferring a darkened area. In three to five days, the fever lowers and the rash begins to fade.

Complications of measles are rare in the generally healthy child. The most common complication of the measles is pneumonia; however, otitis media (ear infections) and other bacterial infections are common because the measles increases a person's susceptibility to streptococcal bacteria.

Personal Protection

Even with lifelong immunity to rubeola, universal precautions are in order. Gloves and washing hands should offer sufficient protection. Wearing a mask and goggles might be appropriate if contact with the patient's respiratory secretions is likely. If you have not had the measles, the current vaccine will offer long-lasting immunity but that immunity is not lifelong. Initial and subsequent vaccinations are suggested.

MUMPS (EPIDEMIC PAROTITIS)

Nature and Spread of the Disease

Mumps is a viral disease characterized by painful swelling of the salivary glands, particularly the parotid glands. It is more prevalent in late winter and early spring. The virus is spread by droplet infection or by direct contact with an object contaminated with the infected person's saliva. The incubation period ranges from 12 to 26 days, and the virus may be present in the exposed person's saliva from 1 to 6 days prior to any swelling of the salivary glands. A person is considered contagious from 1 to 2 days before symptoms appear or after the symptoms disappear. The disease lasts from 5 to 9 days. One episode of the mumps will provide lifelong immunity even though the episode may have been mild or virtually unnoticed.

Signs and Symptoms

After the incubation period, the patient may complain of fatigue, weakness, chills, and have a low-grade to moderate fever before the enlargement of the salivary glands is present. The patient may also complain of pain with chewing or swallowing. Particular discomfort may be reported with swallowing of acidic liquids including fruit juices. As the parotid salivary glands swell, the fever can increase to 104 degrees. The neck beneath the jaw may also swell if other salivary glands become infected. Maximum swelling of the salivary glands occurs by the second day. The disease is short lived and, after 24 to 72 hours, the fever resolves.

Complications of the mumps are rare; however, mumps in the older child, especially those who are past puberty, can have serious effects. Some older boys have experienced inflammation and swelling of a testicle (usually only one side) and some older girls have developed swelling of an ovary (usually only one side). Although sterility can occur in the affected testicle or ovary, hormone production is not affected.

Other complications associated with the mumps include pancreatitis, prostatitis, nephritis, mastitis, and arthritis. Most of these symptoms resolve on their own without lasting effects.

Personal Protection

Having had the mumps as a child will provide immunity if coming into contact with a contagious child. Universal precautions are appropriate as is washing hands because contact with the patient's saliva can result in exposure through direct contact. Vaccinations are available and strongly advised for those without immunity.

CROUP (LARYNGOTRACHEOBRONCHIOLITIS)

Nature and Spread of the Disease

Croup is defined as an acute inflammation of the airways causing inspiratory stridor, seal-bark cough, and respiratory distress. It is not caused by one entity but may be caused by any number of viruses resulting in an upper respiratory infection. Typical causative agents include parainfluenza viruses, respiratory syncytial virus, influenza viruses, and other viruses including the measles. Most often, outbreaks of croup occur in the fall, winter, and spring, and are associated with outbreaks of the various respiratory viruses. Transmission of the disease is by droplet infection or direct contact.

Signs and Symptoms

Prior to the onset of croup, the child usually has a history of recent upper respiratory infection. The nature of the illness is characterized by swelling of the upper airways along with increased airway secretions causing the seal-bark cough and inspiratory stridor. The child awakens at night with spasms of coughing and may develop indications of respiratory failure including rapid, shallow breathing, retraction of the accessory muscles of breathing, and cyanosis. Fever may be present; however, it may be low grade.

The illness generally lasts from three to four days. Mild cases are generally treated at home whereas severe cases will require hospitalization.

Personal Protection

Because croup can be caused by a variety of viruses, use personal protective equipment including gloves and mask. If there is a substantial risk of splashing or contact with the patient's secretions, goggles may be in order. With influenza viruses among the causative agents, getting a flu shot at the beginning of flu season may offer you increased protection against the flu virus that may have caused croup in the patient.

EPIGLOTTITIS

Nature and Spread of the Disease

Epiglottitis is a rapidly developing bacterial disease usually caused by the bacteria *Hemophilus influenzae (H. influenzae).* Occasionally, a streptococcus bacteria may be responsible for the condition, but this is rare. Typically, children over the age of two years are affected; however, the disease can develop at any age, even in adults. The disease can be transmitted to susceptible individuals by droplet infection or by direct contact.

Signs and Symptoms

The disease has a rapid onset and presents with a sore throat, hoarse voice, and fever. Respiratory distress develops quickly and is characterized by dyspnea, dysphagia (difficulty swallowing), aphasia (not speaking), drooling, rapid breathing, and inspiratory stridor. The patient will often assume a tripod position to aid in breathing. In this position, the child sits bolt upright with his hands on the seat of the chair. The child raises his shoulders to ease his breathing by lifting the shoulders upward. With rapid swelling of the epiglottis blocking the airway, the work of breathing often increases. If the epiglottis is irritated by direct visualization of the airway or the child's crying, it can swell further, leading to a fatal blockage of the airway.

A complication of *H. influenzae* bacteria is pneumonia. Additionally, the infection can spread to the joints, meninges, or pericardium, although these complications are rare.

Personal Protection

Most healthy adults are resistant to the bacteria, which have been found as one of the normal bacteria of the mouth and throat. Personal protective equipment including gloves, mask, and goggles is appropriate if advanced airway procedures are required. Hand washing is essential to prevent exposure by direct contact. A vaccine is available for individuals who are susceptible to the bacteria.

RESPIRATORY SYNCYTIAL VIRUS (RSV)

Nature and Spread of the Disease

Respiratory syncytial virus (RSV) is a common cause of respiratory infection occurring in infants and young children. The virus has also been known to cause infection in adults who are repeatedly exposed to infected children. Infections in adults, however, are much milder. The virus is responsible for a variety of conditions ranging from the cold to severe respiratory infection and is most prevalent during the winter months. The disease has occasionally been known to be fatal, especially in the very young or very old. It is transmitted by droplet infection as well as direct and indirect contact.

Signs and Symptoms

The incubation period as well as the signs and symptoms of the illness will be varied depending upon the age and overall health of the patient. The condition can range in severity from a mild cold to pneumonia with signs and symptoms as equally varied. Among the signs and symptoms are dyspnea, coughing, and wheezing, which can appear a few days after the initial signs and symptoms of the infection. Most mild to moderate infections resolve on their own without medical attention or hospitalization.

Personal Protection

Reducing the risk of contracting RSV is best achieved by wearing gloves and, if appropriate, mask and goggles. Hand washing is also essential to avoid transmitting the virus by direct contact. There is no known vaccine to prevent infection.

WHOOPING COUGH (PERTUSSIS)

Nature and Spread of the Disease

Whooping cough is a highly contagious bacterial disease. It causes a spasmodic cough that ends in the characteristic high-pitched whooping sound on inspiration. It is prevalent among young children, usually under the age of two years. Although having the disease does not give lifelong immunity, subsequent attacks are usually milder. Whooping cough is transmitted by droplet infection during the early stages of the disease, when the patient has a runny nose and paroxysms of coughing.

Signs and Symptoms

After an incubation period of from 7 to 14 days, the bacteria invades the mucous membranes of the airways causing an increased production of mucus. The disease can last approximately six weeks and consists of three stages. The initial stage consists of sneezing, watery eyes, loss of appetite, and listlessness. The patient develops a cough that is most noticeable at night, developing into day and night coughing as the disease progresses.

The second stage develops in 10 to 14 days and is characterized by paroxysms of coughing. The paroxysms consist of 5 to 15 rapid consecutive coughs. These coughs are followed by a high-pitched, whooping sound caused by a hurried and deep inhalation. After a few normal breaths, the paroxysm can repeat. With the paroxysms of coughing, thick mucus can be expelled from the airways. The patient may also vomit as a result of the paroxysms of coughing or due to gagging on the mucus.

The third stage begins in approximately four weeks. The paroxysms of coughing decrease in frequency. Residual paroxysms of coughing can last for several months, gradually ending.

Although the mortality rate from whooping cough is extremely low, complications including pneumonia can develop. With increased pressures inside the chest, pneumothorax can develop along with subcutaneous emphysema. Convulsions are possible as well as bleeding into the brain from prolonged paroxysms and associated lack of oxygen.

Personal Protection

With the advent of immunization against the disease, the incidence of pertussis has decreased. However, a young child with whooping cough may still need treatment. Universal precautions—gloves, mask, and goggles—are appropriate. If the patient coughs up substantial amounts of mucus, a gown may be needed to prevent contamination of clothing with infectious material. Thorough hand washing is required. After transportation of the patient, thorough decontamination of the ambulance and equipment is appropriate.

POLIOMYELITIS

Nature and Spread of the Disease

Poliomyelitis, also known as polio or infantile paralysis, is decreasing in prevalence due to intensive efforts in vaccinating children. In third world countries with poor sanitation and no vaccination programs, the incidence of the disease is still high. Polio is caused by a virus transmitted through droplet infection, direct contact, and indirect contact. The risk of exposure by droplet infection is small because the virus has a short life span outside the body. Direct contact with the mucous membranes of the infected individual is the most common mode of transmission although indirect exposure by contact with the patient's blood or feces is also possible. The patient is considered contagious for about seven days from the onset of the disease.

Signs and Symptoms

There are two types of polio—paralytic and nonparalytic. In both cases, the disease begins with fever, headache, vomiting, sore throat, pain and stiffness in the back and neck, and sleepiness. In nonparalytic polio, the fever subsides in approximately seven days and the stiffness resolves in three to five days. In paralytic polio, the signs and symptoms of muscle weakness or paralysis are present within one to seven days of the disease's onset. Weakness or paralysis of the muscles of breathing, swallowing, or speaking usually presents within the first three days of the disease. An early indication of the involvement of these muscles includes dysphagia (difficulty swallowing), nasal regurgitation, and nasal intonation of the voice.

With paralytic forms of the disease, the residual disability varies. Less than 25 percent of patients with paralytic polio have severe disabilities whereas another 25 percent have mild or minimal disabilities. Most patients, however, have no residual effects.

Personal Protection

With the advent of polio vaccines, the incidence of polio in developed countries is minimal. Unfortunately, undeveloped countries are not as fortunate. Immigrants or visitors from third world countries may have the disease when they enter the United States. For those who have been vaccinated against polio, there is little concern about exposure to the disease. However, gloves, mask, goggles, and gown may be appropriate depending on the patient's secretions or the risk of contamination from blood or feces. Hand washing is, as always, essential as is thorough decontamination of the ambulance after transporting an infected patient.

DIPHTHERIA

Nature and Spread of the Disease

Diphtheria is a bacterial disease of childhood that is highly contagious. It affects the membranes of the throat and, in rare instances, other organ systems of the body. If not identified and treated promptly, the disease can be fatal. The diphtheria bacteria is transmitted by droplet or by indirect contact. Droplets from the mouth, nose, and airways of the infected person can spread the disease even after the patient has recovered. Touching or using eating utensils or other objects previously used by the patient can transmit the disease. Diphtheria can also affect the skin through an open wound.

Signs and Symptoms

After an incubation period of from two to five days, the patient will complain of a sore throat, fever, headache, and nausea. The bacteria produces a toxin that destroys the tissues. A false membrane or pseudomembrane forms over the damaged tissue. This pseudomembrane develops in patches and appears gray to dirty-yellow. The size of the pseudomembrane may mislead people about the severity of the infection. In many cases, the infection tends to be deeper and wider than suspected. The toxin can be absorbed by the blood and transported to the heart, nervous system, and kidneys. Unless treatment is prompt and the patient receives the diphtheria antitoxin, the patient can develop myocarditis followed by heart failure and sudden death.

Complications of the disease include swelling of the neck, pharynx, and larynx. If the pharynx or larynx are significantly swollen, the edema can obstruct the airway. In addition, pseudomembranes may be present in the lower airways that could impede airflow or, if the membrane detaches, completely occlude the airway. Other complications include myocarditis and nervous system degeneration.

Personal Protection

In developed countries, childhood immunization against diphtheria protects against this highly contagious bacteria. When treating a patient with diphtheria, wearing gloves, mask, goggles, and a protective garment will impede spread of the disease by indirect contact. Disinfect the ambulance thoroughly after transporting an infected patient and wash hands thoroughly.

CONJUNCTIVITIS (PINKEYE)

Nature and Spread of the Disease

Conjunctivitis, also known as pinkeye, is a highly contagious inflammation of the lining of the eyelids. Viruses, bacteria, and allergies have been known to cause conjunctivitis. For viral and bacterial conjunctivitis, transmission of the disease is usually through indirect contact—touching a contaminated object then rubbing the eyes. Many children develop conjunctivitis and then spread the illness to their parents through close contact.

Signs and Symptoms

Typically, the affected eye or eyes will be reddened or inflamed. The infected eye will have large amounts of mucus secretions that become crusty when dried. The patient will complain of a burning or itching sensation. All vision is normal. Conjunctivitis readily responds to antibiotic therapy and resolves with treatment.

Personal Protection

Because bacterial and viral conjunctivitis are highly contagious, use extreme caution when handling contaminated clothing or other items. Wearing gloves and washing hands should be sufficient protection against infection. If infection occurs, seek prompt medical attention and do not rub the eyes. If the affected eye is rubbed, be sure to wash hands thoroughly before touching anything else, especially the unaffected eye.

IMPETIGO

Nature and Spread of the Disease

Impetigo is a superficial skin infection caused by streptococcus or staphylococcus bacteria. The infection most commonly appears on the arms, legs, and face. Spread of the infection is through direct contact with the moist, infectious material on the skin. If it is not properly treated, the disease can spread between individuals. For newborn infants, impetigo can be fatal.

Signs and Symptoms

Impetigo is characterized by small to large pustules (pus-containing lesions) surrounded by reddened skin. These pustules can rupture, releasing the infectious material. A crust soon forms after the pustule ruptures. The infection causes itching that when scratched can spread the disease to other areas of the body. In the ulcerative form of the disease, small, punched-out ulcers with darkened crusts form on the skin. These ulcers are surrounded by reddened skin.

Treatment consists of applying an antibiotic ointment and isolation in cases where the patient's hygiene is poor. Usually, the most serious consequence of impetigo, particularly ulcerating impetigo, is scarring. However, cellulitis, inflammation of the lymph vessels, and boils on the skin can occur.

Personal Protection

Crusted skin lesions should be considered impetigo and precautions taken not to spread the disease. Gloves are indicated when handling the patient. If it appears that contamination of clothing is possible through contact with the patient, wearing a gown is also suggested. Properly dispose of any contaminated equipment or supplies and disinfect surfaces that were in contact with the patient. Thoroughly wash hands before leaving the hospital.

ROTAVIRUS

Nature and Spread of the Disease

A common cause of diarrhea in infants and children is the *rotavirus,* a wheel-shaped virus that causes approximately 55,000 hospitalizations in the United States each year. The virus is considered extremely contagious and is primarily spread by fecal-oral contact. It has been known to survive on contaminated clothing and toys for several days. Ingestion of contaminated food or water has also been known to result in infection. Rotavirus is most common in the fall and winter months.

Signs and Symptoms

The signs and symptoms of infection can range from mild to severe beginning about two days after exposure. Signs and symptoms include vomiting and watery diarrhea lasting from three to eight days. Infected children will have a fever and often complain of abdominal pain. Complications of the illness are associated with dehydration and problems with the body's electrolytes.

☎ YOU MAKE THE CALL

You arrive at a private residence and are greeted by a frantic woman who claims that her four-year-old daughter is having trouble breathing. She hurriedly escorts you to the kitchen of the house where you find the child in apparent respiratory distress. The girl is sitting bolt upright, leaning slightly forward. Her hands are placed flat on the chair seat and appear to be elevating her shoulders. Her jaw is jutting forward and she is drooling. Inspiratory stridor is noted. Although the girl doesn't speak or respond to your questions, her mother tells you that she was complaining about a sore throat not too long ago.

What do you think may be the cause of the child's distress?

How can this infection be spread to others?

Because this illness is typically seen in childhood, are you at risk for infection?

On another call, you are greeted by a woman who claims that her six-year-old son is ill and itching quite a bit. Upon examining the child laying on his bed you observe that he is covered with a rash on his chest and abdomen. The rash appears to have a red, flattened base with a raised, fluid-filled vesicle. The child is trying hard not to scratch the rash. The woman tells you that the neighbor's child came down with chickenpox and she deliberately sent her son to play at the neighbor's house. You believe that child has contracted chickenpox.

Because you had chickenpox as a child, are you at risk for contracting the disease as an adult?

If you did not have chickenpox as a child, how could you protect yourself against the virus?

Personal Protection

The disease is common in childhood and, once contracted, there is a limited immunity to future episodes. Universal precautions are essential to prevent the spread of the disease to others. Wash hands thoroughly and disinfect any contaminated equipment or clothing. A vaccination is available for children. Consult a pediatrician for more information about the vaccination against *rotavirus*.

SUMMARY

Childhood diseases are highly contagious but pose only a minimal risk for EMTs and paramedics. The risk of exposure to and infection by an infectious agent has been significantly reduced through childhood immunization programs. Many adults have contracted these diseases as children and have developed an acquired, lifelong immunity. Awareness of these diseases and taking precautions will prevent inadvertently transmitting them to others.

Many childhood diseases are viral in nature. However, several illnesses are bacterial. Chickenpox, measles, German measles, mumps, croup, respiratory syncytial virus, and poliomyelitis are caused by viruses. Epiglottitis, whooping cough, and diphtheria are bacterial in nature. Although patients recover from most of these illnesses spontaneously, there are some complications that are known to be life threatening.

Using personal protective equipment—gloves, mask, goggles, and gowns—re-

duces transmission of these diseases. Along with using personal protective equipment, washing hands after contact with each patient helps reduce the risk of infection. Vaccination when available, also serves to reduce chances of infection.

As was mentioned earlier in this chapter, the Advisory Committee on Immunization Practices (ACIP), the American Academy of Pediatrics (AAP), and the American Academy of Family Physicians (AAFP) have developed recommendations concerning childhood immunizations. The Immunization Action Coalition has developed a chart on the Summary of Rules for Childhood Immunization based upon the recommendations of the ACIP, AAP, and AAFP. The chart on the following two pages describes these rules for immunizations for diphtheria, tetanus, pertussis (DTP or DT and Td); Polio (inactive polio vaccine—IPV, or oral polio vaccine—OPV); Varicella (Var), measles, mumps, rubella (MMR); H. influenza (Hib); Hepatitis B (HBV); and rotavirus (Rv). The American Academy of Pediatrics does warn that this information should not be used as a substitute for the care and advice of a pediatrician.

In July, 1999, the Centers for Disease Control and Prevention (CDC) issued a statement recommending that pediatricians not immunize infants against rotavirus. The advisory statement was based upon a report of adverse reactions among infants receiving the vaccine. The press release stated, "CDC recommends that health care providers and parents postpone use of the rotavirus vaccine for infants, at least until November 1999, based on early surveillance reports of intussusception (a type of bowel obstruction that occurs when the bowel folds in on itself) among some infants who received rotavirus vaccine. Although intussusceptions occur among infants who have not received rotavirus vaccine, CDC will be collecting additional data in the next several months that may indicate more clearly whether the rotavirus vaccine increases the risk of intussusception." (CDC Press Release, July 15, 1999)

The press release also contained information on the problem stating, "The rate of intussusception among children receiving the rotavirus vaccine appears to be increased in the first 2–3 weeks after vaccination. Parents and caretakers of infants should contact their health care provider if the child develops symptoms of intussusception (persistent vomiting, bloody stools, black stools, abdominal bloating or severe colic pain). Health care providers should be aware of the possible increased risk and consider this diagnosis among children presenting these symptoms."

Since this measure is temporary and may be revised toward the end of 1999, contact a pediatrician or CDC for additional information.

In related news, the Advisory Committee on Immunization Practices (ACIP) has recommended against the use of the oral polio vaccination (OPV) beginning in January, 2000. This recommendation is based on the incidence of polio caused by the oral vaccine which uses live viruses. (Morbidity and Mortality Weekly Report, July 15, 1999) ACIP does recognize the occasional need for OPV and makes the following suggestions:

"OPV should be used only for the following special circumstances:

1. *Mass vaccination campaigns to control outbreaks of paralytic polio.*
2. *Unvaccinated children who will be traveling in <4 weeks to areas where polio is endemic.*
3. *Children of parents who do not accept the recommended number of vaccine injections. These children may receive OPV only for the third or fourth dose or both; in this situation, health-care providers should administer OPV only after discussing the risk for vaccination associated paralytic polio with parents or caregivers."*

For additional information, contact a pediatrician.

The chart starting on page 42 contains a synopsis of the signs, symptoms, and personal protective equipment for the various childhood diseases.

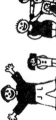
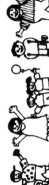

Summary of Rules for Childhood Immunization*

Adapted from ACIP, AAP, and AAFP by the Immunization Action Coalition, March 1999

Vaccine	Ages usually given, other guidelines	If child falls behind—minimum intervals	Contraindications (Remember, mild illness is not a contraindication.)
DTaP contains acellular pertussis **DTP** contains whole-cell pertussis Give IM	• DTaP is preferred over DTP for all doses in the series. • Give at 2m, 4m, 6m, 15-18m, 4-6yrs of age. • May give #1 as early as 6wks of age. • May give #4 as early as 12m of age if 6m has elapsed since #3 and the child is unlikely to return at age 15-18m. • If started with DTP, complete the series with DTaP. • Do not give DTaP or DTP to children ≥7yrs of age (give Td). • DTaP/DTP may be given with all other vaccines but at a separate site. • It is preferable but not mandatory to use the same DTaP product for all doses.	• #2 & #3 may be given 4wks after previous dose. • #4 may be given 6m after #3. • If #4 is given before 4th birthday, wait at least 6m for #5. • If #4 is given after 4th birthday, #5 is not needed. • Don't restart series, no matter how long since previous dose.	(DTaP and DTP have the same contraindications and precautions.) • Anaphylactic reaction to a prior dose or to any vaccine component. • Moderate or severe acute illness. Don't postpone for minor illness. • Previous encephalopathy within 7 days after DTP/DTaP. • Unstable progressive neurologic problem. **Precautions:** The following are precautions not contraindications. Generally when these conditions are present, the vaccine shouldn't be given. But, there are situations when the benefit outweighs risk so vaccination should be considered (e.g., pertussis outbreak). • Previous T ≥ 105°F (40.5°C) within 48 hrs after dose. • Previous continuous crying lasting 3 or more hours within 48 hrs after dose. • Previous convulsion within 3 days after immunization. • Previous pale or limp episode, or collapse within 48 hrs after dose.
DT Give IM	• Give to children <7yrs of age if the child has had a serious reaction to the "P" in DTaP/DTP, or if the parents refuse the pertussis component. • DT can be given with all other vaccines but at a separate site.	For children who have fallen behind, use information in box directly above.	• Anaphylactic reaction to a prior dose or to any vaccine component. • Moderate or severe acute illness. Don't postpone for minor illness.
Td Give IM	• Use for persons ≥7yrs of age. • A booster dose is recommended for children 11-12yrs of age if 5yrs have elapsed since last dose. Then boost every 10 years. • Td may be given with all other vaccines but at a separate site.	For those never vaccinated or behind, of if the vaccination history is unknown: give dose #1 now; dose #2 is given 4wks later; dose #3 is given 6m after #2; and then boost every 10 years.	• Anaphylactic reaction to a prior dose or to any vaccine component. • Moderate or severe acute illness. Don't postpone for minor illness.
Polio **IPV** and **OPV** Give IPV SQ or IM Give OPV PO	• Give at 2m, 4m, 6-18m, and 4-6yrs of age. • Give IPV for doses #1 and #2 (except in special circumstances), e.g., parent's refusal, imminent travel to polio-endemic area). • ACIP says for dose #3, give OPV at 12-18m, and for dose #4, give OPV at 4-6yrs. An all-IPV schedule is also acceptable. If an all-IPV or all-OPV schedule is used, dose #3 may be given as early as 6m of age. • AAP/AAFP say give either IPV or OPV for doses #3 and #4. Dose #3 is given at 6-18m of age and dose #4 at 4-6yrs. • ACIP/AAP/AAFP say IPV is acceptable for all 4 doses. • Not routinely given to anyone ≥18yrs of age (except certain travelers). • IPV may be given with all other vaccines but at a separate site. • OPV may be given with all other vaccines.	• #1, #2, & #3 (IPV or OPV) should be separated by at least 4wks. • All IPV: a 6m interval is preferred between doses #2 and #3 for best response. • #4 (IPV or OPV) is given between 4-6yrs of age. • If #3 of an all-IPV or all-OPV series is given at ≥4yrs of age, dose #4 is not needed. • Children who receive any combination of IPV and OPV doses must receive all 4 doses, regardless of the age when first initiated. • Don't restart series, no matter how long since previous dose.	• Anaphylactic reaction to a prior dose or to any vaccine component. • Moderate or severe acute illness. Don't postpone for minor illness. • Use IPV when an adult in the household or other close contact has never been vaccinated against polio. • In pregnancy, if immediate protection is needed, see the ACIP recommendations on the use of polio vaccine. **The following are contraindications for OPV (so use IPV in these situations):** • Cancer, leukemia, lymphoma, immunodeficiency, including HIV/AIDS. • Taking a drug that lowers resistance to infection, e.g., anti-cancer, high-dose steroids. • Someone in the household has any of the above medical problems.
Varicella **Var** Give SQ	• Routinely give at 12-18m. • Vaccinate all children ≥12m of age including all adolescents who have not had prior infection with chickenpox. • If Var and MMR (and/or yellow fever vaccine) are not given on the same day, space them ≥28d apart. • Var may be given with all other vaccines but at a separate site.	• Do not give to children <12m of age. • Susceptible children <13yrs of age receive 1 dose. • Susceptible persons ≥13yrs of age receive 2 doses 4-8wks apart. • Don't restart series, no matter how long since previous dose.	• Anaphylactic reaction to a prior dose or to any vaccine component. • Moderate or severe acute illness. Don't postpone for minor illness. • Pregnancy, or possibility of pregnancy within 1 month. • If blood, plasma, or immune globulin (IG or VZIG) were given in past 5 months, see ACIP recs or AAP's *1997 Red Book* (p. 353) re: time to wait before vaccinating. • Immunocompromised persons due to high doses of systemic steroids, cancer, leukemia, lymphoma, immunodeficiency. **Note:** For patients on high doses of systemic steroids or for patients with leukemia, consult ACIP recommendations. **Note:** Manufacturer recommends "no salicylates" for 6wks following this vaccine.

* Hepatitis A, influenza, pneumococcal, and Lyme disease vaccines are indicated for many children and teens, so make sure you provide these vaccines to at-risk children. The newer combination vaccines are not listed on this table but may be used whenever administration of any component is indicated and none is contraindicated.

Read the package inserts. For full immunization information, see recent ACIP statements published in the *MMWR*; and for the latest recommendations of the AAP's Committee on Infectious Diseases, see the AAP's *1997 Red Book* and the journal, *Pediatrics*.

Item #P2010 (rev 3/99)

Summary of Rules for Childhood Immunization (continued)

Vaccine	Ages usually given, other guidelines	If child falls behind—minimum intervals	Contraindications (Remember, mild illness is not a contraindication.)
MMR Give SQ	• Give #1 at 12-15m. Give #2 at 4-6yrs. • Make sure that all children (and teens) over 4-6yrs have received both doses of MMR. • If a dose was given before 12m of age, give #1 at 12-15m of age with a minimum interval of 28d between MMR #1 and MMR #2. • If MMR and Var (and/or yellow fever vaccine) are not given on the same day, space them ≥28d apart. • May give with all other vaccines but at a separate site.	• 2 doses of MMR are recommended for all children ≤18yrs of age. • Give whenever behind. Exception: If MMR and Var (and/or yellow fever vaccine) are not given on the same day, space them ≥28d apart. • There should be a minimum interval of 28d between MMR #1 and MMR #2. • Dose #2 can be given at any time if at least 28d have elapsed since dose #1, and both doses are administered after 1 year of age. • Don't restart series, no matter how long since previous dose.	• Anaphylactic reaction to a prior dose or to any vaccine component. • Pregnancy or possible pregnancy within next 3m (use contraception). • Moderate or severe acute illness. Don't postpone for minor illness. • If blood, plasma, or immune globulin were given in past 11 months, see ACIP recs or *1997 Red Book* (p. 353) re: time to wait before vaccinating. • HIV is NOT a contraindication unless severely immunocompromised. • Immunocompromised persons, e.g., cancer, leukemia, lymphoma. Note: For patients on high-dose immunosuppressive therapy, consult ACIP recommendations regarding delay time. Note: MMR is NOT contraindicated if a PPD test was done recently, but PPD should be delayed if MMR was given 1-30 days before the PPD.
Hib Give IM	• HibTITER (HbOC) & ActHib (PRP-T): give at 2m, 4m, 6m, 12-15m. • PedvaxHIB (PRP-OMP): give at 2m, 4m, 12-15m. • Dose #1 of Hib vaccine may be given as early as 6wks of age but not earlier. • May give with all other vaccines but at a separate site. • All Hib products licensed for the primary series are interchangeable. • Any Hib vaccine may be used for the booster dose. • Hib is not routinely given to children ≥5yrs of age.	**Rules for all Hib vaccines:** • The last dose (booster dose) is given no earlier than 12 months of age and a minimum of 2 months since the previous dose. • For children ≥15m and less than 5yrs who have NEVER received Hib vaccine, only 1 dose is needed. • Don't restart series, no matter how long since previous dose. **Rules for HbOC (HibTITER) & PRP-T (ActHib) only:** • #2 and #3 may be given 4 wks after previous dose. • If #1 was given at 7-11m only 3 doses are needed: #2 is given 4-8wks after #1, then boost at 12-15m. • If #1 was given at 12-14m, give a booster dose in 2m. **Rules for PRP-OMP (PedvaxHIB) only:** • #2 may be given 4 wks after dose #1. • If #1 was given at 12-14m, boost 8wks later.	• Anaphylactic reaction to a prior dose or to any vaccine component. • Moderate or severe acute illness. Don't postpone for minor illness.
Hep-B Give IM	• Vaccinate all infants at 0-2m, 1-4m, 6-18m. • Vaccinate all children 0-18 years of age. • For older children/teens, spacing options include: 0m, 1m, 6m; 0m, 2m, 4m; 0m, 1m, 4m. • Children who were born or whose parents were born in countries of high HBV endemicity or who have other risk factors should be vaccinated as soon as possible. • **If mother is HBsAg positive:** give HBIG and hep-B #1 within 12hrs of birth, #2 at 1-2m, and #3 at 6m of age. • **If mother's HBsAg status is unknown:** give hep B #1 within 12hrs of birth, #2 at 1-2m, and #3 at 6m of age. If mother is later found to be HBsAg-positive, her infant should receive the additional protection of HBIG within the first 7 days of life. • May give with all other vaccines but at a separate site. • Hepatitis B vaccine brands are interchangeable.	• Don't restart series, no matter how long since previous dose. • 3-dose series can be started at any age. • Minimum spacing for children and teens: 4wks between #1 & #2, and 2m between #2 & #3. Overall there must be 4m between #1 and #3. • Dose #3 should not be given earlier than 6 months of age. **Dosing of hepatitis B vaccines:** For Engerix-B, use 10µg (0.5ml) for 0 through 19 yrs of age. For Recombivax HB, use 5µg (0.5ml) for 0 through 19 yrs of age.	• Anaphylactic reaction to a prior dose or to any vaccine component. • Moderate or severe acute illness. Don't postpone for minor illness.
Rota-virus Rv Give PO	• Give at 2m, 4m, and 6m. • Dose #1 should not be given before 6wks or at ≥7m. • No dose should be given on or after the first birthday. • Do not readminister a regurgitated dose. • May give with all other vaccines.	• Minimum interval is 3wks between doses. • Use minimum intervals to achieve protection prior to rotavirus season or if behind schedule. • Don't restart the series no matter how long since previous dose.	• Moderate or severe acute illness, including persistent vomiting. Don't postpone for minor illness. • Anaphylactic reaction to a prior dose or to any vaccine component. • Known or suspected altered immunity, including infants born to HIV+ mothers unless it is known that the child is not HIV infected. • For infants with pre-existing chronic GI conditions, see ACIP statement.

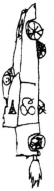

"I follow the rules of the road. If you follow the rules of immunization, you won't get lost!"

The Immunization Action Coalition developed this table to combine the recommendations for childhood immunization onto one page and to assist health care workers in determining the appropriate use and scheduling of vaccines. It can be posted in immunization clinics or clinicians' offices.

Comments? E-mail: nedinfo@immunize.org, call 651-647-9009, or mail to IAC at 1573 Selby Avenue, St. Paul, MN 55104.

Thank you to the following individuals for their review: William Atkinson, MD, Harold Margolis, MD, Linda Moyer, RN, Jane Seward, MBBS, Robert Sharrar, MD, Thomas Vernon, MD, Richard Zimmerman, MD. Final responsibility for errors lies with the editors.

This table is revised yearly. The most recent edition of this table is available on our website at <www.immunize.org>

Disease	Signs/Symptoms	Personal Protection
Chickenpox	Headache	Gloves
	Reduced appetite	Vaccination
	Fever	
	Rash	
	Red, flat discoloration	
	changes to itchy vesicles	
	contains clear fluid	
German measles	Fatigue	Gloves
(Rubella)	Rash	Vaccination
	Red spot with raised area	
	Flushed skin	
	Swollen lymph nodes	
	Fever	
	Headache	
	Joint pain/stiffness	
	Stuffy nose	
Measles	Fever	Gloves
(Rubeola)	Runny nose	Vaccination
	Cough	
	Conjunctivitis	
	Headache	
	Neck pain	
	Sore throat	
	Koplik's spots	
	Rash	
	Small reddened area	
	Raised papule	
	Itching	
Mumps	Fatigue	Gloves
	Weakness	Vaccination
	Fever	
	Chills	
	Swelling of salivary glands	
Croup	History of respiratory infection	Gloves
	Seal-bark cough	Mask
	Inspiratory stridor	Goggles
	Rapid, shallow breathing	if splashing possible
	Retraction of accessory muscles	
	Cyanosis	
Epiglottitis	Rapid onset sore throat	Gloves
	Fever	Mask
	Dyspnea	Goggles
	Difficulty swallowing	if splashing possible
	Drooling	
	Shallow breathing	
	Inspiratory stridor	
	Tripod position	

Disease	Signs/Symptoms	Personal Protection
Respiratory syncytial virus	Mild to severe cold Dyspnea Coughing Wheezing	Gloves Goggles if splashing possible

Whooping cough (Pertussis)	Increased mucus production
	Sneezing
	Watery eyes
	Loss of appetite
	Listlessness
	Paroxysms of coughing
	  5 to 15 rapid, successive coughs
	  followed by whooping sound
	  paroxysms can repeat
		Gloves
		Mask
		Goggles
		  if splashing possible
		Vaccination

Poliomyelitis	Fever
	Headache
	Vomiting
	Sore throat
	Pain and stiffness in neck and back
	Sleepiness
	Paralysis can develop
	  Affects skeletal muscles
	  Difficulty speaking
	  Difficulty breathing
	  Difficulty swallowing
		Gloves
		Mask
		Goggles
		  if splashing possible
		Vaccination

Diphtheria	Sore throat
	Fever
	Headache
	Nausea
	False membrane forms
	  Covers damaged tissue
	  Appears gray or dirty-yellow
		Gloves
		Mask
		Goggles
		Garment

Conjunctivitis (Pinkeye)	Affected eye is inflamed Mucus secretions turning crusty Burning or itching sensation Vision is normal	Gloves

Impetigo	Reddened skin
	Large pustules
	  Can rupture
	  Releases infectious material
	  Pustules crust after rupturing
	Ulcers may form on affected skin
		Gloves
		Garment
		  to protect clothing

5

Coming of Age
Infectious Diseases Found in Adults

OBJECTIVES

At the end of the chapter, the reader will be able to:

1. Define the following terms:

Asymptomatic	Babinski's reflex
Chancre	Gangrene
Hemoptysis	Macule
Purulent	Pustule
Sputum	Vesicles

2. State the modes of transmission, signs, and symptoms of the influenza virus.
3. State why senior citizens are high risk with the regard to the flu.
4. State the modes of transmission, signs, and symptoms of meningitis.
5. List three signs or symptoms of tuberculosis.
6. Discuss the use of personal protective and vehicle equipment used when treating or transporting patients with pulmonary tuberculosis.
7. List the signs or symptoms of necrotizing fasciitis.
8. List three sexually transmitted diseases and their signs and symptoms.
9. Understand that unnecessary and excessive use of antibiotics have led to the creation of antibiotic-resistant bacteria.

In the preceding chapter, we reviewed common childhood diseases that EMS professionals may encounter. Most EMTs and paramedics are at a reduced risk for contracting a childhood illness such as measles, mumps, or rubella, because they have either had the disease as a child or been vaccinated against it. But EMS personnel are still at risk of exposure to serious or life-threatening illnesses every time they respond to a call. Although not all patients put EMTs and paramedics at risk for serious illness, there are a few that harbor dangerous bacteria or viruses.

This chapter focuses on the more common infectious diseases encountered in the prehospital setting. Diseases range from influenza, causing mild discomfort, to tuberculosis that can cause a fatal infection. Although hepatitis, HIV, and AIDS are included in these diseases, this book devotes separate chapters to discussing each one of those illnesses. This chapter focuses on the flu, impetigo, meningitis, tuberculosis, necrotizing fasciitis, and several sexually transmitted diseases.

WORDS TO KNOW

Asymptomatic meningitis   A condition when the meninges are inflamed, but no infectious agent can be found.

Asymptomatic   Having no signs or symptoms of a disease.

Babinski's reflex   An abnormal response in people over 18 months of age, seen when the sole of the foot is scraped. The response is characterized by the upward flexion of the big toe and fanning out of the remaining toes. It indicates abnormalities in the central nervous system.

Chancre   A papule found in syphilis that breaks down into an ulcer. It is characterized by little if any pain.

Crepitus   Caused by air in the tissues, palpation of the affected area creates a "popping" sound.

Debridment   The removal of foreign material or damaged tissues from an infected area until normal, healthy tissue is found.

Encephalitis   Inflammation of the brain.

Gangrene   Death of body tissue from loss of blood supply due to damage to or destruction of the blood vessels. Bacterial infection and decomposition of the tissue cause it to turn dark and emit a foul odor.

Hantavirus   A virus spread by rodent droppings causing severe respiratory distress.

Hemophilus influenzae   A bacteria that can cause meningitis.

Hemoptysis   Coughing blood.

Hemorrhagic bronchitis   Inflammation of the bronchi and bronchioles causing bleeding.

Herpes simplex virus   A virus that causes fluid-filled blisters to erupt on the skin. The blisters can be oral or genital.

Herpes zoster   The virus that causes chickenpox invades the nervous system and, after many years of being dormant, causes pain, fever, vesicles and pustules on the skin.

Immunocompromised   Characteristic of a person whose immune system has been weakened and cannot resist infection by bacterial or viral agents.

Impetigo   An infection of the skin caused by streptococcus or staphylococcus bacteria.

Kyphosis   Abnormal curvature of the spine often referred to as hunchback.

Macule   A discolored spot on the skin that is not raised or elevated.

Meninges   The three coverings of the brain and spinal cord.

Meningitis   Inflammation of the meninges.

Meningococcus   A bacteria that causes some cases of meningitis.

Mycobacterium tuberculosis   Bacteria responsible for most cases of tuberculosis.

Myocarditis   Inflammation of the heart muscle.

Oro-genital contact   Contact with the genitals by the mouth.

Purulent   Containing or forming pus.

Pustule   A small, elevated lesion of the skin that contains pus.

Sputum   A mucus secretion of the airways that is coughed from the lungs and expelled through the mouth.

Tubercles   Small, rounded areas consisting of fibrous tissue used to wall off an infection.

Vesicles   Small elevations of the skin containing fluid.

INFLUENZA

Nature and Spread of the Disease

The common flu or influenza is an upper respiratory disease caused by a virus typically seen during the fall and winter. Widespread influenza cases are reported primarily in winter months. Two main types of influenza viruses cause the upper respiratory infection: type A and type B. A lesser studied type C is also responsible for infections in adults. Although type A is the most common cause of influenza, both strains of the virus have been known to cause serious and occasionally fatal illness. Type C influenza has been known to cause mild respiratory disease.

The virus is spread by direct contact with an infectious person, airborne contamination by infected droplets, or indirect contact with contaminated surfaces such as drinking glasses, eating utensils, towels, and discarded infectious garbage.

Signs and Symptoms

The disease is typically characterized by fever, runny nose, cough, inflammation of the airways, generalized aches, and it has an incubation period of 48 hours. The onset of the illness is rapid, initially presenting with weakness and aches and pain usually in the back and legs. Headache is also common. Chills brought on by a fever between 102°F and 103°F develop within the first 24 hours of the illness. With the onset of the flu, the respiratory system may be mildly affected, usually with a sore throat and dry cough. A runny nose may also be present. As the disease progresses, the cough becomes productive and can become severe. In some cases, hemorrhagic bronchitis and pneumonia can develop. The acute phase of the disease generally lasts two to three days but can endure as long as five days.

Most people who contract the flu recover without any problems, although complications can develop. High-risk persons—including the elderly, patients with compromised immune systems, and those with chronic heart or lung conditions—may develop pneumonia, hemorrhagic bronchitis, or a secondary bacterial infection. If the fever, cough, and other respiratory signs and symptoms continue for more than five days, pneumonia or a secondary, bacterial infection should be suspected. Other complications associated with influenza include myocarditis and encephalitis.

Personal Protection

Individuals who have had the flu are immune to that same flu virus for a short period of time. The best protection against influenza is vaccination. Although the vaccine cannot provide complete immunity from all the variations of the virus, it does offer protection from the known or prevalent strains of the disease. Vaccination is highly recommended for high-risk patients and those at substantial risk for contracting the disease.

Universal precautions will reduce but not eliminate the chance of infection. Gloves are essential when handling infectious materials, and if the patient has a severe and productive cough, wearing a mask and gown will reduce the risk of exposure. Because EMS professionals will be exposed to the flu, EMTs and paramedics are urged to receive an annual flu vaccine.

IMPETIGO

Impetigo was discussed in the chapter on childhood diseases. Because it can be transmitted to adults, a brief review is in order. Impetigo is a skin infection caused by either streptococcus or staphylococcus bacteria. It is transmitted by direct contact with an infectious person.

Signs and symptoms of the disease include vesicles that become pustular and rupture, forming yellow crusts. Scratching of the infected area can lead to the spread of the disease to other parts of the body or to other people. A form of the disease called ecthyma causes ulcerations that appear to be small, purulent ulcers with a thick brown-black crust.

Using universal precautions, especially gloves when touching the patient, will help prevent spread of the disease. Wear a gown or protective garment to protect your clothing, and properly dispose of linens and decontaminate exposed equipment. Finally, wash hands thoroughly after any contact with patients.

HERPES ZOSTER—SHINGLES

Nature and Spread of the Disease

Shingles is a contagious viral disease that is caused by the same virus as chickenpox. It is primarily an infection of the nervous system, characterized by eruption of vesicles on the skin as well as pain and itching. After exposure to and infection with the chickenpox, the virus enters the sensory nerves and travels to the nerve roots where it becomes dormant for many years. People who are infected generally do not show any signs or symptoms of infection. The disease can become activated by any number of factors including stress, fatigue, cancer therapy, and the use of drugs to suppress the immune system.

It is estimated that over 10 percent of the adult population who had chickenpox as a child will develop shingles later in life. Although shingles can affect anyone at any age, it usually affects people over the age of 50.

Although the disease is less contagious than chickenpox, it can be transmitted by direct contact with the vesicles. People who have not been vaccinated against chickenpox or have not had chickenpox are at risk.

Complications of shingles include continued muscle weakness, which, in most cases, will spontaneously disappear. For some, the pain associated with the disease persists for a while after the infection has cleared. A person with a weakened immune system or one who is malnourished may be at risk for a secondary infection of the vesicles, which could lead to tissue destruction and scarring.

Signs and Symptoms

The disease progresses in stages. The initial onset of the illness is characterized by fever and chills accompanied by weakness and fatigue. A person may complain of pain or skin sensitivity in the areas where the vesicles will appear. Occasionally, the patient may complain of abdominal or chest pain, which could be mistaken for another condition. Approximately four to five days after the initial signs and symptoms, the vesicles appear and continue appearing for up to a week. The vesicles usually appear on the chest and spread to one side of the body; however, they can appear anywhere. Eventually, the vesicles turn into pustules, rupture, and crust.

Personal Protection

As with chicken pox, universal precautions are important. Gloves are essential and a gown should be worn if clothing may come in contact with the patient. Wash hands immediately after caring for the patient. In most cases, one episode of shingles will give the person a lifelong immunity; however, recurrent attacks do occur. EMTs and paramedics who have not had the chickenpox are urged to be vaccinated against the disease.

EPIGLOTTITIS

Nature and Spread of the Disease

Although this disease is more commonly found in children (as discussed in the last chapter), it can also be seen in adults and pose a life-threatening emergency. It is important to discuss epiglottitis in this chapter on diseases of adulthood. Epiglottitis is a rapidly developing bacterial disease usually caused by the bacteria *Hemophilus influenzae (H. influenzae)*. A streptococcus bacteria may be responsible for the condition, but this is rare. Primarily, children over the age of two years are affected; however, the disease can develop at any age, even in adults. The disease can be transmitted to susceptible individuals by droplet infection or by direct contact.

Signs and Symptoms

The disease has a rapid onset and presents with a sore throat, hoarse voice, and fever. Respiratory distress develops quickly and is characterized by dyspnea, dysphagia, aphasia, drooling, rapid breathing, and inspiratory stridor. The patient will often assume a tripod position to aid in breathing. With rapid swelling of the epiglottis blocking the airway, the work of breathing often increases. If the epiglottis is irritated by direct visualization of the airway, it can swell further, leading to a fatal blockage of the airway.

A complication of *H. influenzae* bacteria is pneumonia. Additionally, the infection can spread to the joints, meninges, or pericardium although these complications are rare. These complications can be seen in adults and children.

Personal Protection

Most healthy adults are resistant to the bacteria that causes epiglottitis. It is one of the normal bacteria of the mouth and throat. Personal protective equipment including gloves, mask, and goggles is appropriate if advanced airway procedures are required. Hand washing is essential to prevent exposure by direct contact. A vaccine is available for individuals who are susceptible to the bacteria.

MENINGITIS

Nature and Spread of the Disease

Meningitis is the inflammation of the coverings of the brain and spinal cord (meninges). The inflammation can be either viral or bacterial. Viral meningitis can be contracted from a prior viral infection such as the mumps, measles, rubella, or another virus. Many cases of viral meningitis are postinfections—they originate from another primary infection. Often, no infectious agent can be identified in viral meningitis. That is why it is called aseptic meningitis.

Bacterial meningitis is caused by several bacteria including *Neisseria meningitidis* (meningococcus), *Hemophilus influenzae,* and pneumococcus. Transmission of the infectious agent is through direct contact with the mucous membranes of the infected person. Droplet infection also poses a risk of transmission. For the bacteria to cause meningitis, it must have a portal of entry into the central nervous system. Head trauma is one cause. The bacteria also may have entered the bloodstream through the mucous membranes of the upper airways.

Recently, new strains of bacteria causing meningitis have been discovered. Some of these new strains are resistant to antibiotics. A common antibiotic, chloramphenicol, is used to treat meningitis in many areas of the world because it is abundant and inexpensive. However, new strains of *Neisseria meningitidis* have been identified, and studies indicate that the genetic mutation allowing for drug resistance is easily spread to other strains of *N. meningitidis.*

Signs and Symptoms

Bacterial meningitis has a sudden onset after a respiratory illness caused by one of the offending infectious agents. Typically, the patient will complain of an intense headache, fever, nausea, vomiting, and a stiff neck. The patient may also be lethargic, delirious, or comatose and may present with seizures. The patient may have a rash caused by a systemic infection that led to the meningitis. In a patient with a stiff neck, sudden flexion of the neck will result in the involuntary flexion of the hips and knees. Some patients may demonstrate Babinski's reflex on one or both feet. Another indication of meningitis is known as Kernig's sign. A patient laying supine can extend his or her legs. However, if a leg is flexed toward the abdomen, the patient cannot extend or straighten the knee.

Because bacterial meningitis can be fatal in a matter of a few hours, anyone suspected of the infection should be immediately transported to the appropriate emergency department. Even with prompt recognition and treatment, the mortality rate of meningitis ranges between 5 and 10 percent. If untreated, up to 50 percent of the victims of meningitis will die. Additionally, between 15 and 20 percent of disease survivors will have some residual central nervous system problem such as deafness or mental retardation.

Personal Protection

Because transmission of the disease is through direct contact with mucous membranes or droplet infection from airborne secretions, universal precautions, particularly gloves, are important. Use a mask and goggles if contamination from airborne respiratory secretions is likely. Clean or dispose of any infectious or contaminated materials appropriately.

A vaccination against some forms of bacterial meningitis *(N. meningitidis)* is available. If it is not obtainable for a particular type of infectious agent, preventive therapy is available following exposure. Antibiotics such as rifampin have been prescribed to counter potential infection.

TUBERCULOSIS

Nature and Spread of the Disease

Tuberculosis is caused by bacteria known as *Mycobacterium tuberculosis* and other types of mycobacteria such as *M. kansasii* and a new agent, *Mycobacterium canettii.* Tuberculosis is an airborne disease transmitted by inhaling dried or moist droplets of infectious material coughed up or sneezed by the patient. The incidence of tuberculosis is currently increasing throughout the world, especially in developing nations. Tuberculosis is also increasing in the United States particularly among the homeless, migrants, and HIV-positive patients. Lax public health measures or preventive programs including screening, vaccinations, and treatment have allowed the increase of tuberculosis. An associated dilemma is that new strains of tuberculosis are being identified that are resistant to antibiotics.

The most common site of infection is the lung; however, other areas of the body can be infected. These include the spine or other bony areas, meninges, kidneys, liver, and spleen.

Two types of infection are involved with tuberculosis: primary and secondary. Primary tuberculosis is seen as an initial infection. This infection is small and usually resolves with no further spread of the disease. A secondary infection can be a reactivation of a prior infection or a reunification. When a person's health declines due to any number of causes, the infection can reactivate and spread throughout the body.

After infection and an incubation period of from 4 to 12 weeks, tubercles form. These tubercles consist of fibrous tissue to wall off the infection. With a small infection in a person whose health status is good, the infection is controlled and possibly eliminated. In immunocompromised patients or patients whose health status is weakened, the infection can spread throughout the lungs and to other organs. Small granulomas or tubercles can spread through the organ, eventually resulting in organ failure.

Signs and Symptoms

The patient with tuberculosis will present like many other patients with infectious diseases—fever, chills, weakness, and night sweats. The patient will experience weight loss and have complaints of shortness of breath (dyspnea) and a productive cough. The sputum often appears green to yellow in color. As the disease progresses, the sputum will contain blood (hemoptysis). Eventually, the patient with pulmonary tuberculosis will develop respiratory failure.

With the spread to other organ systems, associated signs and symptoms will appear. For example, in spinal or bony tuberculosis, the disease is usually found in the thoracic or lumbar spine and, eventually, the knee and hip. With spread to the bone, there is extensive necrosis of the tissue leading to compression fractures and a hunchback appearance (kyphosis).

Personal Protection

Universal precautions and respiratory isolation are important. To transport a patient with tuberculosis, remove any unnecessary equipment prior to responding to the call. Have the patient wear a nonporous mask if he or she is not in respiratory distress or failure. Use a nonporous mask yourself and keep the patient away from other EMS personnel. Use the ventilation fan in the patient compartment at all times the patient is onboard your ambulance. Finally, thoroughly disinfect your vehicle prior to restocking or responding to another call.

Periodic testing by a PPD skin test as offered or mandated by your employer is essential for early detection of the disease. If a PPD test is positive, further evaluation by a physician, a chest X-ray, and prophylactic antibiotics are the usual course of action.

NECROTIZING FASCIITIS (FLESH-EATING STREP)

Nature and Spread of the Disease

The media have recently caused alarm over what they label "Flesh-Eating Strep." According to the media, people are dying from or becoming severely disfigured as a result of the treatment for the disease. Necrotizing fasciitis is a reality although its prevalence is infrequent. The disease is caused by a mixture of various streptococcus bacteria, some of which thrive in oxygen-free environments whereas others require oxygen to survive. The bacteria cause damage by entering the skin through an open wound. The wound, which is often small or minor, can be caused by blunt or open trauma, chemical or thermal burns, and even surgical trauma.

Once the bacteria have invaded the skin, they can cause tissue swelling and death to subcutaneous tissues. Blockage of the smaller blood vessels enhances the tissue destruction and can lead to gangrene. The bacteria that thrive without oxygen produce hydrogen and nitrogen gases that accumulate under the skin causing crepitus. The end result of the infection is death of the tissue.

Signs and Symptoms

The predominate complaint is severe pain at the site of the infection. The skin over the infected tissue is flushed, hot, and swollen. As the disease progresses, the skin will become discolored, fluid-filled blisters will appear, and gangrene develops. The patient will have a fever and, if the entire body is involved, may present with altered mental status.

The mortality rate of necrotizing fasciitis is high, approaching 30 percent. Some patients at risk of death are the elderly and those with underlying medical conditions such as diabetes. Although antibiotic therapy is helpful, the most effective treatment includes extensive debridment including amputation if needed.

Personal Protection

Wearing gloves is essential. Even more critical is washing the hands with soap and water. As mentioned above, the wound allowing the bacteria to invade the body does not have to be large. Cover and protect breaks in the skin and use antimicrobial ointments to prevent infection. If any clothing or linens contact the patient, dispose of properly.

HANTAVIRUS

Nature and Spread of the Disease

Hantavirus has recently received increased media attention due to deaths it has caused. Also known as hemorrhagic fever, the virus is found in the Southwestern United States and has also been identified in other parts of the country as well as throughout the world. Although it is not a widespread or common illness, the potential severity of the disease does attract attention, particularly through a severe form of the illness known as hantavirus pulmonary syndrome (HPS).

Hantavirus is a virus that resides in rodents such as mice and rats where it poses no problems for its host. Rat and mouse droppings, including feces and urine, have been known to harbor the virus. Even when dried, the virus can be transmitted to people by dustborn particles. The virus has not been transmitted from person-to-person.

Signs and Symptoms

After infection, the initial stages of the illness have been described as non-specific meaning that they cannot be easily associated with any particular disease. During the early stage of the illness, the patient will have a fever and complain of aches and pains. The patient may also complain of headaches, nausea, vomiting, abdominal pain, diarrhea, cough, and general weakness. As the disease progresses, the patient may develop severe shortness of breath, dizziness, sweats, and chest or back pain. Once this later stage begins, the patient's condition is critical, requiring hospitalization and assisted ventilation due to respiratory failure and pulmonary edema.

Personal Protection

In an open area where droppings are few and dust minimal, gloves will suffice. In a closed area, where droppings are numerous and contaminated dust could be disturbed, a face mask or respirator may also be necessary. Be sure to disinfect any equipment and thoroughly wash hands after contact with the patient.

EMTs and paramedics are not, as a rule, at risk for sexually transmitted diseases while on duty. However, some sexually transmitted diseases can be transmitted via modes other than sexual relations. Bloodborne transmission or transmission via direct or indirect contact can spread herpes, syphilis, and chlamydia. This section of the chapter discovers some of the sexually transmitted diseases that could pose a risk. This section does not discuss gonorrhea, trichomoniasis, candidiasis, or genital warts.

Herpes

Nature and spread of the disease.   Herpes has been given considerable media attention for the version that is sexually transmitted—genital herpes. The genitals are just one location of many where herpes can erupt.

Herpes is a viral infection caused by the herpes simplex virus. It can appear anywhere on the skin or mucous membranes and is most frequently seen on the mouth, lips, conjunctiva, cornea, and genitals. After the initial infection, which is often unknown, the virus invades the body and resides in the nerve ganglia until a trigger mechanism activates the infection and causes vesicles to erupt. Although the trigger mechanism for a specific eruption is usually unknown, they can include stress, overexposure to the sun, some foods and drugs, and a weakened immune system.

The virus is spread via direct contact with a vesicle. Touching the lesion with the fingers or lips can spread the virus to another person. Oral contact via kissing can also transmit the disease. Oro-genital contact can spread the virus from a cold sore to the genitals. Newborns can also become infected during the birth process when they contact vaginal lesions.

Signs and symptoms.   During the initial stages of the eruption, there is some mild discomfort including itching and tingling at the site. Shortly thereafter, small vesicles appear either singly or in clusters. The eruption may be painful in tender areas or when it is associated with underlying structures such as the nose, ear, or fingers. After a few days, the vesicles begin to dry and heal, forming a yellow crust. The eruption usually starts to heal within 8 days and is complete within 21 days. In genital herpes, the lesions are considerably more painful. The vesicles erode and form small ulcerations that crust a few days after appearing. Healing occurs in about 10 days.

Complications associated with herpes, particularly genital herpes, include aseptic meningitis (see above) and problems with the functions of the autonomic nervous system.

Personal protection.   When examining a patient with herpes, universal precautions, including gloves, are appropriate. Washing hands after patient contact is essential. If a woman with genital herpes is in labor, wearing gloves, masks, goggles, and protective garments is appropriate. Any reusable equipment that has been in contact with the patient should be disinfected thoroughly.

Syphilis

Nature and spread of the disease.   Syphilis is caused by the bacteria *Treponema pallidum,* a spiral organism that is very fragile and cannot live for very long outside of the body. The bacteria enters the body usually during sexual intercourse, but it can be transmitted by contact with an open lesion (chancre). Occasionally, the disease is transmitted by kissing or close physical contact where the bacteria can enter the body through minute abrasions in the skin. Once inside the body, the bacteria travel to regional lymph nodes and are spread throughout the body. The circulatory and central nervous systems are infected during the early stages, and, if left untreated, syphilis causes significant arterial and central nervous system damage.

Signs and symptoms.   After entering the body, the incubation period averages from three to four weeks and appears in stages. There are three main stages of untreated syphilis: the primary stage, a secondary stage followed by a latent period, and a tertiary or late stage.

In the primary stage, following the incubation period, a chancre appears at the site where the bacteria entered the body. The chancre initially appears reddened and raised, soon forming a painless ulcer. If bumped or contacted, the ulcer does not bleed. The bacteria are present in a clear fluid that spreads the disease to others. Chancre sores can be found in a number of places including the genitals, anus, fingers, mouth, lips, tongue, and tonsils. Because the chancre is painless, it is often ignored. The chancre will spontaneously heal.

In 6 to 12 weeks after becoming infected, the secondary stage of syphilis develops. This stage is characterized by a rash that appears as macules, papules, or pustules that are generally painless and do not itch. Eventually, the rash will disappear, leaving no scars. Lymph nodes in the neck, armpit, and other palpable areas become enlarged but are not painful.

The next stage of syphilis is the latent stage, during which the patient appears normal. In approximately one-third of the patients, the disease disappears completely. In others, the latent stage has no associated signs or symptoms, yet the bacteria are still present for many years.

After the latent period, about half of the remaining infected patients will develop the late or tertiary stage of syphilis. During this stage, benign, noninfectious lesions appear on the body and can appear on the skin, subcutaneous tissues, and mouth. Although the lesions can appear anywhere on the skin, they are more prevalent below the knees. Not only do the lesions develop on the skin and subcutaneous tissues, they can also develop on internal organs including the stomach, liver, lung, and other structures.

Cardiovascular syphilis and neurosyphilis can develop. Cardiovascular syphilis is characterized by an aneurysm of the ascending aorta. In neurosyphilis, the patient can be asymptomatic or can show signs of dementia, including changes in behavior, loss of or difficulty speaking, weakness on one side of the body, and convulsions.

Personal protection.   A patient with syphilis cannot readily be identified. Some patients have been diagnosed with the disease and may be receiving treatment. When examining a patient with syphilis, universal precautions including gloves are appropriate. After examining and touching the patient, it is essential that the EMS professional wash his or her hands. If a woman is in labor, wear gloves, masks, goggles, and gown or suit to protect against splashing or contamination of face and clothing from the patient's body fluids. Any reusable equipment that has been in contact with the patient should be disinfected thoroughly.

Chlamydia

Nature and spread of the disease.   Chlamydia is a rapidly spreading, sexually transmitted disease. The Centers for Disease Control and Prevention estimate that over 4 million new cases of chlamydial infection develop each year. But chlamydia is not merely a sexually transmitted disease. It can be spread to others during nonsexual contact and it can infect organs including the respiratory system.

Chlamydia is caused by the bacteria *Chlamydia trachomitis*. Although most of the media attention has been given to the sexually transmitted disease, chlamydia can be responsible for infections in other areas of the body such as the eyes. *Chlamydia trachomitis* has been identified in lower respiratory infections.

In genital chlamydial infections in men, the bacteria cause inflammation of the urethra, epididymis, and rectum. In women, inflammation of the cervix and fallopian tubes is common. Rectal inflammation can also occur. Transmission of the bacteria can occur during vaginal, oral, or anal sexual contact with the infected person. Chlamydia can also be transmitted from an infected mother to her newborn during childbirth.

The disease can be spread to other areas of the body, particularly the eyes. Infectious secretions on the fingers or hands can be transmitted by direct contact to the eyes, resulting in conjunctivitis. Indirect contact can also occur when contaminated objects are in contact with mucous membranes of the body. For example, an eyeliner or mascara brush contaminated with chlamydia can result in an infection to the eyes. Contaminated towels used to dry the face can also spread the disease to the eyes. Respiratory infection is more common in immunocompromised patients; however, its spread to people with normal immune systems is increasing.

Signs and symptoms. Genital chlamydia may be difficult to identify. It is often mistaken for gonorrhea and frequently coexists with a gonorrhea infection. The signs and symptoms of chlamydia develop after a one- to three-week incubation period. In many men and women (estimates are 25 percent of men and 75 percent of women), there are no symptoms and it may not be diagnosed until complications develop. In women, signs and symptoms include an abnormal discharge from the vagina or urethra along with pain or a burning sensation during urination. The vaginal opening may be inflamed, and bleeding may present after sexual intercourse. In later stages, the woman may complain of lower abdominal pain and abnormal vaginal bleeding. In men, signs and symptoms include an abnormal discharge from the urethra and painful urination. If the disease spreads to the epididymis, pain is present with palpation of the tissue around the testes. The discharge is either clear, white, or yellow.

Complications of genital chlamydia infections include swelling of the lymph nodes in the groin. This can lead to inflammation of the rectum in men and narrowing of the rectum in women. If untreated, this can lead to fever and pain in the joints. Eventually, rectal narrowing and drainage occurs.

Chlamydial infections of the eyes result in conjunctivitis characterized by a purulent discharge from the eyes. Complications of chlamydial infections to the eyes can include scarring of the conjunctiva and blindness.

Personal protection. As with herpes and syphilis, protection consists of using universal precautions including gloves, mask, goggles, and gown when appropriate. Thoroughly wash hands and discard or dispose of contaminated linens properly. Disinfect contaminated equipment following your agency's protocols.

A vaccine had been developed in hopes of reducing the risk of transmission and spread of the disease. Studies have shown that the vaccine failed to halt the disease, and in those who received the vaccine, the disease is more severe.

THE MEGABUGS!

Media-grabbing headlines warn of the dangers of Ebola, anthrax, or biologic warfare. What the media fail to warn about are the new drug-resistant strains of bacteria and viruses. What can be considered the same old bug has a brand new package, and some of the more powerful antibiotics are unable to stop its spread. Consider, for example, a strain of staphylococcus known as MRSA. MRSA is the acronym for Methicillin Resistant Staphylococcus Aureus. MRSA is being seen with increasing frequency in hospitals and skilled nursing facilities. Because this infection is resistant to the standard antibiotics, treatment with a more powerful antibiotic, Vancomycin®, is required.

There is a strain of staphylococcus that is resistant to the more powerful antibiotics including Vancomycin. Whereas cases of the Vancomycin-resistant bacteria have been limited to the Far East, reports in the literature have discussed cases of Vancomycin-resistant staphylococcus infection appearing in the United States. Information can be found on these specific megabugs in the following section.

In 1985, reports appeared in the news media revealing that drug-resistant bacteria and viruses pose a serious threat to health. Initial reports said officials from the CDC have found bacterial infections that cannot be treated with any of the known or currently used antibiotics.

These sentiments have been echoed by experts around the world. Reports from various conferences and numerous articles state that resistance to even the most powerful antibiotics is increasing. Some bacteria have been reemerging with a strong resistance to many available antibiotics. Vancomycin-resistant *Staphylococcus aureus* has been reported in Japan and in the United States. There have even been reports of drug-resistant tuberculosis, especially in HIV-positive patients.

Some of the reasons behind the emergence of drug-resistant bacteria are as follows:

Unnecessary use of antibiotics. Taking an antibiotic for a viral infection is ineffective, and existing bacteria can change into a strain of bacteria that are not affected by the medication. Patients should not receive an antibiotic for a cold unless there is a bacterial cause or secondary infection for that cold.

Antibiotics may have been inappropriately prescribed. Giving the wrong medication or an inappropriate dose allows the bacteria to alter form or mutate, providing resistance to later administration of medications. Usually, a bacterial infection is cultured in a laboratory and subjected to the medications that can destroy it. In some cases, doctors may prescribe a drug not knowing if that drug will destroy the infection. If the medication is not or only partially effective, the bacteria could mutate and become totally resistant to the drug.

Nonmedical use of antibiotics. Antibiotics used in farming, such as tetracyclines given to livestock as growth promoters, have hastened antibiotic resistance.

EMS professionals need to be aware that new strains of infectious agents are developing. In addition, newly emerging diseases are being reported continually. Awareness of these new hazards will help protect you from exposure. EMS personnel also need to realize the importance of universal precautions in protecting against unwanted and potentially dangerous infections.

Nature and spread of the disease. Methicillin Resistant Staphylococcus Aureus (MRSA) is a staphylococcus bacteria that has, over the years, become resistant to many of the antibiotics that formerly destroyed it. With widespread use of antibiotics in hospitals and skilled nursing facilities, the bacteria have developed a resistance to the once-powerful drugs used to eradicate it. Drugs such as methicillin, penicillin, nafcillin, cephalosporin are no longer effective in treating MRSA. Currently, MRSA infections, once diagnosed, are treated with Vancomycin. Unfortunately, reports indicate that a newer strain of staphylococcus—Vancomycin-resistant staphylococcus aureus—is appearing.

The bacteria are spread between patients usually by health-care workers who come in contact with an MRSA-infected patient and pick up the bacteria on their hands or clothing. The primary mode of transmission is by the EMT or paramedic's own hands after touching a patient without personal protective equipment. If the EMT or paramedic has an MRSA infection, he or she can transmit the bacteria to a patient when in contact with the patient.

After the MRSA infection has been diagnosed, treatment consists of more powerful antibiotics such as Vancomycin. However, as just mentioned, certain strains of staphylococcus are becoming resistant to this powerhouse of an antibiotic.

Signs and symptoms. The signs and symptoms of an infection depend upon the site of the infection. If MRSA infects an open wound, signs of the infection such as skin pustules, redness, swelling, and pain will be present. At times, staphylococcus is present on the skin with no indication of infection. In other infections, the patient may have an infection of his circulatory system or have pneumonia. Thus, it is difficult to determine the nature and presence of MRSA in any given patient.

Personal protection. At a minimum, gloves should be used whenever in contact with a patient suspected of having MRSA. It is also important to wash hands immediately after removing gloves and prior to performing other duties. If performing procedures in which splatter or splashing with body fluids is possible, wear a face mask and protective eyewear such as goggles. If physical contact with the patient or contaminated bed linens or clothing is possible, or if body fluid splashing is likely, also wear a gown or protective garment.

Some extra precautions are in order when preparing to transport a patient with MRSA. After placing the patient on the stretcher, cover the patient with a disposable sheet and tuck the sheet gently under the patient. Remove soiled gloves and replace with clean gloves. When moving the stretcher and patient through any hallway, be sure not to contaminate paperwork or parts of the facility such as countertops or walls.

After transporting the patient, clean any reusable patient care equipment using a disinfectant solution. Any disposable items, including linen, should be placed in a red biohazard bag and properly discarded.

Vancomycin-Resistant Enterococcus (VRE)

Nature and spread of the disease. The bacteria known as enterococcus are normally found in the intestines and, as such, rarely pose any problems. There are a multitude of strains of enterococci bacteria living inside the body.

The strain that is resistant to Vancomycin is known as Vancomycin-Resistant Enterococcus (VRE).

The bacteria have been described as not very harmful unless they invade other areas of the body such as the urinary tract or circulatory system. Infections in these areas can be severe and, at times, life threatening. Healthy individuals are rarely at risk for infection with VRE; however, those with health problems or weakened immune systems could more easily be infected.

VRE is typically found in hospitalized patients or those receiving care in a skilled nursing facility. The bacteria are spread by direct contact with a patient's feces. An EMS professional called to care for a patient with bowel incontinence could come in contact with the patient's feces and inadvertently transmit the bacteria to another patient. Similarly, contaminated surfaces such as cabinets or medical instruments including blood pressure cuffs and stethoscopes could transmit the bacteria.

Personal protection. Universal precautions such as gloves are essential when assessing and treating a patient with VRE. A gown should be worn if patient care will involve physically touching the patient to move him or her for treatment or transportation. Be sure to disinfect all contaminated surfaces such as the stretcher and any medical equipment immediately after transporting the patient. Prior to responding to another call, be sure to wash the hands thoroughly. Although healthy people are at minimal risk for VRE, EMS professionals can spread the disease to other patients if precautions are overlooked.

☎ YOU MAKE THE CALL

You respond to a migrant labor camp where you are escorted into a cramped, one-bedroom apartment. You find five adults and six children sitting on mattresses strewn about the floor. The adults point to a corner of the room where you see a middle-aged man leaning against a wall. As you approach, the man begins to cough violently and produces a bloody mucus that he spits into a paper bag next to him. A brief examination reveals a thin male in respiratory distress. In questioning the man, along with the other adults in the apartment, you learn that the man has had a fever and night sweats with difficulty breathing for the past several months. Over the last few days he has seemed to be getting worse. The others are worried that the man could have pneumonia from the flu that has been going around.

Based upon your overall evaluation of the situation, what condition do you suspect in this case?

What precautions would you take to avoid exposure to the infectious disease while on the scene?

What precautions would you take while transporting the man to the emergency department?

After the call is over, what could you do to determine if you have been exposed to the man's infection?

SUMMARY

This chapter has reviewed many of the infectious diseases that you may encounter in the prehospital setting. Information has been presented on viral and bacterial infections such as the flu, impetigo, meningitis, tuberculosis, and flesh-eating strep. Although it is unlikely that you will be at substantial risk for many of these diseases, you should be aware of potential risks when responding to a call for help.

This chapter also presented information on certain sexually transmitted diseases. Even though you will not be at risk for a sexual transmission of the infectious agent, some of these viruses and bacteria can be transmitted in nonsexual ways. By being alert to the possibility of contracting a disease that is usually sexually transmitted, you can avoid or reduce the risk of exposure. In essence, the phrase "Know your enemy" is very important.

Finally, this chapter touched on the emerging megabugs, or drug-resistant bacteria and viruses that are starting to be identified. Without the ability to fight the new variations of bacteria or viruses, their spread may go unchecked. The chart on the following pages is included for a quick reference of the signs, symptoms, and personal protective equipment for the various diseases seen in adults.

Disease	Signs/Symptoms	Personal Protection
Influenza (Flu)	Fever	Gloves
	Runny nose	Mask
	Cough	Garment
	Inflamed airways	Vaccination
	Generalized aches	
	Weakness	
Impetigo	Reddened skin	Gloves
	Large pustules	Garment
	Can rupture	to protect clothing
	Releases infectious material	
	Pustules crust after rupturing	
	Ulcers of skin may form	
Herpes zoster (Shingles)	Fever, chills	Gloves
	Weakness, fatigue	Garment
	Sensitive or painful skin	To protect clothing
	Vesicles	Vaccination
	Turn into pustules	
	Can rupture	
	Release Varicella virus	
	May have residual pain	
Epiglottitis	Rapid onset sore throat	Gloves
	Fever	Mask
	Dyspnea	Goggles
	Difficulty swallowing	If splashing possible
	Drooling	
	Shallow breathing	
	Inspiratory stridor	
	Tripod position	

(continued)

Disease	Signs/Symptoms	Personal Protection
Meningitis	Sudden onset	Gloves
	History of respiratory infection	Mask
	Severe headache	Goggles
	Fever	if splashing possible
	Nausea and vomiting	Vaccination
	Stiff neck	
Tuberculosis	Fever	Gloves
	Chills	HEPA mask
	Weakness	Or respirator
	Night sweats	Garment
	Weight loss	Use exhaust fan in vehicle
	Shortness of breath	PPD skin test
	Productive cough	
	Green/yellow mucus	
	Blood may be present	
Necrotizing fasciitis	History of open injury	Gloves
(Flesh-Eating Strep)	Severe infection at wound site	Wound care
	Tissue is flushed, hot, swollen	Antibiotic ointment
	Blisters	
	Gangrene	
Herpes	Itching and tingling at site	Gloves
	Appearance of small vesicles	If woman in labor
	May be tender or painful	Mask
	Will dry and form crust	Goggles
	May erode and form ulcers	Garment
Syphilis	Chancre (initial stage)	Gloves
	Painless	If woman in labor
	Does not bleed	Mask
	Rash (second stage)	Goggles
	Macules/papules	Garment
	Painless	
	Does not itch	
	Lymph nodes enlarged	
	Lesions (third stage)	
	Skin and internal organs	
	Painless	
	Altered mentation if CNS involved	
Chlamydia	May be asymptomatic	Gloves
	Abnormal vaginal discharge	If woman in labor
	Abnormal discharge from penis	Mask
	Painful urination	Goggles
	Conjunctivitis if eyes infected	Gown

When the Food Comes Back to Bite You!
Food Poisoning

OBJECTIVES

At the end of the chapter, the reader will be able to:

1. Define the following terms:

Antitoxin	Botulism
Enterohemorrhagic	Gastroenteritis
Incubation	Spores

2. List the signs and symptoms of salmonella food poisoning.
3. List the signs and symptoms of *E. coli* food poisoning.
4. List the signs and symptoms of staphylococcal food poisoning.
5. List the signs and symptoms of botulism poisoning.

Not only are EMTs and paramedics at risk from viruses and bacteria in the air they breathe or in a patient's blood, they can also be exposed to foodborne pathogens—the food we bite can bite back. Media hype, particularly associated with recent incidents of tainted food products, has brought more attention to the hazards in the foods we eat.

There are four bacteria we need to consider as causes of food poisoning. These bacteria are salmonella, *E. coli,* staphylococcus, and *Clostridium botulinum.* The purpose of this chapter is to discuss these bacterial agents and the causes, signs, symptoms, and prevention of bacteria-induced food poisoning.

WORDS TO KNOW

Antitoxin A particular kind of antibody produced to fight or neutralize the effects of a toxin or poison.

Clostridium botulinum A toxin-producing bacteria that causes the life-threatening effects seen in botulism food poisoning.

Enterohemorrhagic From the words *entero* meaning intestine and *hemorrhage* meaning bleeding, the word means intestinal bleeding.

Escherichia coli (pronounced esh'e-rik' e ah) The bacteria *E. coli*—one of many commonly found in the intestines. A variant of this bacteria can cause severe food poisoning.

Gastroenteritis Inflammation of the lining of the stomach and intestines. Signs and symptoms include severe abdominal pain, nausea, vomiting, and diarrhea.

Incubation The time from the invasion of a pathogen into the body until the signs and symptoms appear. This time allows for the growth and spread of the organism.

Intestinal motility The ability of the intestines to move its contents, typically through peristalsis.

Salmonella A type of bacteria that can cause food poisoning. There are many types of salmonella bacteria including one that causes typhoid fever.

Salmonellosis Infection with the species of the salmonella bacteria that causes food poisoning.

Spores In cases of botulism, the spore is considered the resting stage in the life of the bacteria. It is resistant to environmental changes.

Staphylococcus An infectious organism that resides on the skin and in the upper respiratory system. It causes a wound that generally discharges pus.

Ulceration A process of inflammation that destroys a local part of the inner lining of an organ.

SALMONELLA

Nature and Spread of the Disease

A very common form of food poisoning comes from salmonella bacteria, typically found in tainted animal products. The bacteria have a number of variations including the strain that causes typhoid fever. With salmonella, there is a range of infections from gastroenteritis presenting with diarrhea, abdominal cramps, and fever, to the systemic, life-threatening typhoid fever requiring antibiotic therapy. The most common form of salmonella infection is the one that causes acute but self-limiting gastroenteritis. An estimated 2 million cases of salmonella food poisoning occur in the United States annually.

Salmonella bacteria, with the exception of the typhoid variation, requires an animal host reservoir, meaning that animals, including people, can carry the bacteria. Contamination can be found in fowl (chickens and turkeys), pigs, and cattle. We contract the disease when we eat uncooked or underprepared foods such as beef, chicken, or eggs and those foods that contain a sufficient number of salmonella bacteria. Even cooked beef that has not been refrigerated can harbor the bacteria in sufficient numbers to cause salmonellosis.

Most of the bacteria enter the body through the gastrointestinal system when contaminated food is ingested. Once the bacteria have survived the stomach acids, they pass into the intestines and invade the lining of both the small and large bowel. As they invade the bowel, the bacteria produce toxins that inflame the intestines, leading to abdominal pain or cramping along with diarrhea. Although rare, this inflammatory response can lead to ulceration of the bowel and the spread of the bacteria into the blood, allowing for a systemic infection requiring antibiotic treatment.

Signs and Symptoms

Typically, the incubation period for salmonella food poisoning ranges from 6 to 48 hours. The onset of the disease usually takes the form of nausea, followed by vomiting, diarrhea, and abdominal cramps. Muscle aches as well as headache are common complaints. A low-grade fever may also be present. The disease is usually self-limiting and the fever and diarrhea will last for 2 to 7 days.

Treatment

Treatment of the common and self-limiting gastroenteritis includes fluid replacement and controlling pain, nausea, vomiting, and diarrhea. During the course of the disease, the body will respond to eliminate the bacteria in a number of ways including increased intestinal motility (movement), mucus production, and antibody response. Again, it is rare for a systemic infection to occur.

Protecting Yourself

Eliminating salmonella bacteria is difficult because the most common reservoirs harboring the bacteria that infect people are poultry and livestock. Several methods to reduce animal contamination and cross-contamination have been put in place in meat and poultry processing plants. However, we can further reduce our risk of exposure in several ways. First, cook food thoroughly. Raw eggs have been known to contain salmonella bacteria. After handling raw chicken or turkey, wash your hands with soap and water. In addition, disinfect the countertop or cutting board used in preparing the chicken or turkey.

When treating a person with diarrhea from an unknown cause, consider salmonella food poisoning as a possible source. Typically, person-to-person transmission of the disease is unlikely. However, wear gloves and handle soiled linens appropriately. Be sure to wash your hands as well as disinfect areas that were in contact with the patient.

ESCHERICHIA COLI (E. COLI)

Nature and Spread of the Disease

The media have brought another foodborne pathogen to our attention with sensational headlines about undercooked hamburger or tainted fruit drinks causing the hospitalization or death of several children. The pathogen blamed for the problem is *E. coli*. Although *E. coli* is a normal part of the bacteria that inhabit our intestines, the strain that causes the problems reported in the media is different from the one living in human intestines.

The variation of *E. coli* receiving the media attention is a member of the enterohemorrhagic *E. coli* group. As the word implies, it causes bleeding in the gastrointestinal tract. The variant bacteria can be present in the intestines of cattle and spread to the meat during the packing process. In meat processing, slicing beef is generally safe unless contaminated knives or other instruments are used. A contaminated knife will introduce the bacteria into the meat where they can then multiply and pose a risk for infection. When beef is ground, the chance for infection is substantially higher because the bacteria can be spread throughout the beef quickly. Not only can *E. coli* be found in cattle, it can also be found in fruit juices or milk that have not been pasteurized.

The effects of the disease are contingent upon several factors including the number of bacteria consumed, the health status of the person, and the person's resistance to the bacteria's toxin. Young children and the elderly are more susceptible to *E. coli* infection and its effects.

After ingestion, any surviving bacteria can invade the lining of the intestines where they produce toxins, causing inflammation of the tissues and diarrhea. The toxins can damage not only the lining of the bowel, but the blood vessels in the gut, causing gastrointestinal bleeding. If the bacteria invade deeper, they can affect the blood vessels of other organs, particularly the kidneys, and cause bleeding from these organs.

Signs and Symptoms

With infection by *E. coli,* there is an acute onset of watery diarrhea and severe abdominal cramps. The diarrhea becomes bloody within 24 hours of the onset of the infection. A fever may be present but is usually low grade. The diarrhea can last from 1 to 8 days in uncomplicated cases. If a systemic spread occurs and the kidneys are affected, renal failure may develop.

Treatment

Although this form of food poisoning is also self-limiting, the patient should be observed and treated for severe fluid loss, including blood loss. Even though the bacteria can be destroyed by most antibiotics, drug treatment has not been effective in relieving the signs and symptoms of the disease. Hospitalization is suggested for young children or the elderly, especially if complications develop.

Protecting Yourself

Because the most common sources for exposure are in undercooked beef or unpasteurized milk or fruit juices, the simplest way to reduce risk is to cook meats thoroughly, especially hamburger, and drink pasteurized milk or fruit juices. Clean any surfaces that have been in contact with raw meat as well as wash hands thoroughly after handling the raw meat. Transmission of the bacteria from person-to-person is also possible through fecal-oral contact; thus wearing gloves, properly disposing of linens, and washing hands are critical. If the disease is contracted, monitor all diarrhea for the presence of blood and, if seen, contact a doctor as soon as possible.

STAPHYLOCOCCUS

Nature and Spread of the Disease

Staphylococcus bacteria are not only a cause of skin infection; they can also be a source of food poisoning. Staphylococcal food poisoning is caused by the bacteria's toxin rather than the organism itself. The transmission of the infection is usually by food handlers with a staphylococcal infection on their skin. They contaminate the foods they are preparing. These foods, then, are left at room temperature. Foods that are subject to staphylococcal contamination include custards, cream-filled desserts, puddings, dairy products, and processed meats and fish that provide an excellent growth medium in which the bacteria can multiply and produce the toxin.

These foods, which may be available on a buffet table, do not have a spoiled taste. However, the toxins that have been accumulating in the food will cause the gastrointestinal distress typically seen in staphylococcal food poisoning.

Signs and Symptoms

The incubation period for staphylococcal food poisoning is short, usually from two to eight hours after ingesting the contaminated food. The bacteria do not cause the problem because they do not invade the lining of the intestines. The signs and symptoms are caused by the ingested toxins. The onset is quick, heralded by severe nausea and vomiting. The patient may also complain of abdominal cramps, diarrhea, headache, fever, and weakness. In severe intoxication, shock may develop. Complications of staphylococcal food poisoning are generally limited to the very young or very old.

Treatment

Treatment is supportive. Because the disease will last from three to six hours, fluid replacement and monitoring vital signs are all that are necessary. In the unlikely event that shock develops, prompt fluid resuscitation and hospitalization are necessary.

Protecting Yourself

Staphylococcal food poisoning is transmitted from foods that are allowed to sit at room temperature, especially if those foods have been prepared by someone with a skin infection. In a restaurant, it is unlikely that you will know if the food handler has a staphylococcal infection. If unsure, stay away from unrefrigerated foods.

In treating a person with staphylococcal food poisoning, there is no concern for person-to-person transmission. However, applying the universal precautions is appropriate in handling the patient and any soiled linens or patient care items.

BOTULISM

Nature and Spread of the Disease

Botulism received considerable media attention several years ago, and although the hype has quieted, this method of food poisoning has not disappeared. The incidence of botulism food poisoning is quite low, yet it can be fatal. The causative bacteria is *Clostridium botulinum,* particularly its toxin. There are three types of botulism poisoning—foodborne, infant, and wound botulism. Of the three types, the most common is infant botulism followed by foodborne botulism. Because this chapter focuses on food poisoning, it does not discuss wound botulism.

Clostridium botulinum is a bacteria that grows in the soil and produces spores that can remain dormant until conditions allow the bacteria to grow. Most cases of botulism are caused by improper canning of foods. In home canning, preparing a food by exposing it to boiling water does not kill the spores. The spores are heat resistant and will continue to survive after many hours at 100°C (212°F). However, at higher temperatures, especially with moist heat, the spores are destroyed. Thus, poor canning techniques can allow spores to survive and, ultimately, toxins to develop. In contrast to the spores, the toxins will be destroyed at much lower temperatures.

In foodborne botulism, it is the ingestion of the toxins that causes the poisoning. In cases of infant botulism, the infant ingests spores from contaminated foods. Once in the gastrointestinal tract, the bacteria produce the toxins that the body absorbs.

Seven types of toxins are produced by the bacteria, four of which are hazardous to people. When a toxin is ingested, it is absorbed by the body and interferes with the body's nervous system, especially the parasympathetic nervous system. The signs and symptoms for foodborne and infant botulism are similar.

Signs and Symptoms

The onset of botulism is sudden and generally develops within 18 to 36 hours after ingestion. In some cases of foodborne botulism, the incubation period has been from as short as 6 hours to as long as a week or more. The clinical picture of botulism includes constipation as a frequent initial finding, especially in infants. Nausea and vomiting accompanied by abdominal cramps and diarrhea can follow and generally precede neurological signs and symptoms. Neurological signs include descending bilateral weakness or paralysis along with slow heart rate, hypotension, and urinary incontinence. As muscular weakness progresses, difficulty swallowing occurs, often leading to aspiration pneumonia. Respiratory infections can develop, and, with the weakening of the respiratory muscles, respiratory failure can follow.

Treatment

The greatest threat to the patient's life is respiratory failure. Supporting ventilation is critical, and all patients suspected of botulism poisoning should be hospitalized and carefully monitored. Botulism antitoxins are available and, if indicated, should be given as soon as possible after the diagnosis has been made. Although the antitoxins will not reverse existing signs and symptoms, they will slow or stop the progression of the poisoning. With respiratory support and the administration of antitoxin, the survival rate is quite high.

You respond to a call at a private residence where you find a 14-year-old boy complaining of severe stomach cramps. He is nearly immobile on the floor of the bathroom and has had severe diarrhea, which, according to the boy, did have some blood. In questioning the teenager, you learn that he was at an overnight camp the day before with friends. He drank some fresh fruit juice and experienced the first episodes of diarrhea a few hours later. Although he wanted to come home, he felt he should "stick it out" with his friends but the diarrhea was getting worse. The boy tells you that the garbage from the camping trip is in the trash cans in the garage. Your partner returns with the suspected source of contamination—a fresh fruit drink that has not been pasteurized.

What is the common infectious agent suspected in this case of food poisoning?

In addition to nonpasteurized fruit juices, what are some other sources of the bacteria that can cause food poisoning?

Which bacteria are associated with food poisoning originating in raw chicken or eggs?

Which bacteria are responsible for food poisoning from contaminated dairy products?

What can you do to reduce the chances of contracting food poisoning?

Protecting Yourself

Reducing the risk of botulism poisoning includes discarding any canned foods that indicate spoilage. Further, infants less than one year of age should not be fed honey because spores may be present in the honey.

Botulism toxins are biohazards and must be treated as such. Even small amounts of toxin accidentally ingested, inhaled, or absorbed through the eye or a break in the skin can result in a serious illness. All infectious materials from the patient should be handled by specially trained individuals to reduce the chance of contamination. EMS personnel who have not received hazardous materials training should not attempt to handle materials containing the botulism toxin.

SUMMARY

Food poisoning is an uncomfortable disease characterized in most cases by severe abdominal distress, nausea, vomiting, and diarrhea. The signs and symptoms of the diseases are related to the bacteria's effects on the gastrointestinal system or the effects of the toxins produced by the bacteria. In some cases, systemic infection by the bacteria or its toxin can result in life-threatening conditions. Although there are reported deaths from food poisoning, the mortality rate is rather low.

With proper food handling, food preparation techniques, and the use of universal precautions when caring for a patient with food poisoning, we can reduce the number of cases of the disorder and reduce the chance of becoming a victim of the malady. The chart that follows has been included for a quick reference of the signs, symptoms, and personal protective equipment for the various types of food poisoning.

Disease	Signs/Symptoms	Personal Protection
Salmonella	Onset in 6 to 48 hours	Gloves
	Nausea	Goggles
	Vomiting	if splashing possible
	Diarrhea	
	Cramps	
	Muscle aches	
	Headache	
	Low-grade fever	
Escherichia coli	Watery diarrhea	Gloves
(E. coli)	Severe abdominal cramps	
	Bloody diarrhea	
Staphylococcus	Onset in 2 to 8 hours	Gloves
	Nausea	
	Vomiting	
	Abdominal cramps	
	Diarrhea	
	Headache	
	Fever	
	Weakness	
Botulism	Onset in 18 to 36 hours	Biohazardous material
	Nausea	Haz-Mat equipment
	Vomiting	Gloves
	Abdominal cramps	Mask
	Diarrhea	Goggles
	Muscle weakness	Protective suit
	Bradycardia	
	Hypotension	
	Respiratory failure	

Dangerous Acronyms
HIV and AIDS

OBJECTIVES

At the end of the chapter, the reader will be able to:

1. Define the following terms:

   Anorexia   Asymptomatic
   Candidiasis   Cytomegalovirus
   Hemophiliacs   Pelvic inflammatory disease
   Peripheral neuropathy   T-helper cells

2. Understand HIV and AIDS and their effects on the immune system.
3. List risk factors of HIV or AIDS.
4. List the 14 signs and symptoms associated with HIV and AIDS.
5. Describe what is meant by the term *opportunistic infection.*
6. List the opportunistic infections commonly found in patients with AIDS.

In the early 1980s, first reports of a rapidly spreading epidemic began to appear. AIDS was recognized in the United States in 1978 and reported in the professional journals in 1981. The media picked up and followed stories about a sexually transmitted disease that was infecting thousands and perhaps millions of people in the United States and throughout the world. As scientists raced to identify the cause of the infection, an underlying current of panic spread nearly as fast as the disease. With time and study, researchers were able to identify the Human Immunodeficiency Virus (HIV) as the infectious agent and determined how the virus entered and infected the body. They also identified how the virus affects the body, ultimately leading to the condition known as Acquired Immunodeficiency Syndrome (AIDS).

There are many books written about this lethal virus. Continuing research is uncovering more about how to fight the infection and keep it under control. The purpose of this chapter is not to serve as a comprehensive guide to HIV and AIDS. Its purpose is to familiarize EMS professionals with the nature of the disease, how it infects the body, its modes of transmission, and the risk factors for contracting AIDS. We also discuss the Centers for Disease Control and Prevention's (CDC) guidelines for AIDS classification. This chapter presents information on the opportunistic infections that result in the victim's death. Finally, we discuss the signs and symptoms of a person infected with HIV as well as review personal protection against the virus.

WORDS TO KNOW

AIDS   The acronym for Acquired Immunodeficiency Syndrome.

Anorexia   Lack or loss of appetite.

Asymptomatic   Having no signs or symptoms of a disease.

Candida albicans   The infectious agent causing vaginal yeast infections and oral thrush.

Candidiasis   Infection by *Candida albicans*.

Cryptosporidium enterocolitis   Inflammation of the intestines (enterocolitis) by the protozoa cryptosporidium.

Cryptosporidosis   Infection by the protozoa cryptosporidium.

Cytomegalovirus   From the herpes group of viruses, it can result in acute illness characterized by fever and inflammation of the liver and lungs. In those with AIDS, cytomegalovirus can also affect other organs, such as the central nervous system and kidneys. In the final stages of AIDS, patients with cytomegalovirus may have inflammation of the brain along with ulcerations of the esophagus or intestines.

Encephalopathy   A degenerative disease of the brain caused by a number of conditions.

Hemophiliacs   Patients who lack a specific blood-clotting factor and who have a tendency to bleed profusely. Blood products are used to treat the condition.

HIV   The acronym for Human Immunodeficiency Virus.

Kaposi's sarcoma   A malignant tumor that appears blue-red in color. It usually appears on the lower extremities but can spread to other parts of the body, including internal organs.

Lymphadenopathy   Generalized enlargement of the lymph nodes.

Lymphocyte   One of the white blood cells that make up the body's immune system and the precursors of the immune system. Lymphocytes are primarily located in the lymph nodes and lymph-like tissues throughout the body.

Pelvic inflammatory disease   Inflammation of the female pelvis including the uterus, fallopian tubes, and ovaries. The inflammation can extend to other abdominal organs.

Peripheral neuropathy   Deterioration in function of the nerves located in the periphery (arms/hands and legs/feet) of the body. Deterioration could include decreased sensation of pain.

Pneumocystis carinii *pneumonia*   Pneumonia caused by the protozoa *Pneumocystis carinii,* causing severe respiratory distress and respiratory failure.

T-cytotoxic cells   Killer cells—lymphocytes responsible for killing cells bearing a specific kind of antigen.

T-suppressor cells   Lymphocytes that suppress antibody production as well as the production and function of T-helper and T-cytotoxic lymphocytes.

Toxoplasmosis   A protozoa that invades the body and causes cysts to develop in muscle tissue and the vital organs.

NATURE AND SPREAD OF THE DISEASE

The infectious agent in this lethal disease is a virus known as Human Immunodeficiency Virus (HIV). In order to survive, the virus needs to copy or replicate itself by using the host's (patient's) body cells. Once inside the patient, the virus seeks and finds T-helper lymphocytes. As discussed in Chapter 3 on the immune system, the primary function of the T-helper lymphocyte is, as the name implies, to help the immune system, acting as a regulator of the system's functions. To accomplish their job, T-helper cells form different proteins called interleukins and interferons, which stimulate the production of the two other T-lymphocytes known as T-cytotoxic (killer) and T-suppressor cells.

Once HIV is close enough to the T-helper cell, it binds with it and fuses with the cell membrane, releasing its genetic information into the T-helper cell. After releasing the genetic information into the T-helper cell, the virus can replicate itself. In the process of replication, the host cell, the T-helper lymphocyte, is killed. With the T-helper cells damaged or destroyed, they can no longer help the immune system fight infecting agents. Research has also indicated that HIV can infect and destroy other types of cells associated with the immune system including monocytes and macrophages. With the immune system impaired, the patient's natural defenses are inhibited or inactivated.

AIDS is the end stage of the HIV infection and is characterized by single or multiple opportunistic infections. There is a distinct difference between HIV and AIDS. Although HIV infection may have occurred, a person is not considered having AIDS unless he or she has suffered a serious compromise or breakdown of the immune system. Such a compromise is a CD4 count less than 200/cc of blood or the presence of one or more opportunistic infections. A common marker in HIV-positive patients is the CD4 level. CD4 is an antigen found on the surface of the T-helper cells. HIV binds to the CD4 and infects the cell, eventually destroying it. Normally, CD4 levels range from 800 to 1,200 per cc of blood.

Opportunistic infections occur in patients whose immune system is compromised or unable to fight the invasion of bacteria, viruses, and other in-

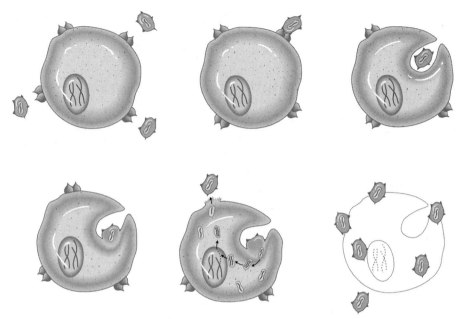

HIV infecting T-helper lymphocyte and replicating itself, destroying the lymphocyte.

fectious agents. They are rarely seen in healthy individuals whose immune systems are functioning normally. With a damaged immune system, these infectious agents have the opportunity to invade, multiply, and infect.

If an HIV-positive person is diagnosed with AIDS and recovers from the opportunistic infection or the CD4 count returns to about 200, he or she will still be diagnosed as having AIDS.

HIV is a fragile virus—it cannot survive for long outside the body. The typical modes of transmission include contact with infected blood or body fluids through sexual contact, sharing contaminated needles, needle-stick injuries, and mother–child transmission. It is not possible to contract HIV from kissing, hugging, casual contact, coughing, sneezing, or sharing meals or eating utensils. It had been thought that the virus was spread through saliva and tears; however, cases of HIV transmission by these routes have not been confirmed. Mosquito and other animal bites have been suspected of transmitting HIV but are not confirmed methods of HIV transmission.

People at high risk for exposure to HIV include homosexual or bisexual men, IV drug abusers, blood transfusion and organ transplant recipients, sex-

STATISTICS

Total cases of HIV/AIDS since start of epidemic	688,200
Total number of people living with HIV/AIDS	372,586
Total number of HIV cases	106,575
Number of new HIV cases 1998 in men	12,698
Number of new HIV cases 1998 in women	5,967
Number of new cases of AIDS in 1997	60,270
Number of new cases of AIDS in 1998	48,269
Number of new AIDS cases 1998 in men	36,886
Number of new AIDS cases 1998 in women	10,998

Source: HIV/AIDS Surveillance Report, Vol. 10, no. 2 (December 1998).

ual partners of men at high risk for the disease, children of high-risk parents, and hemophiliacs. HIV has begun to spread into the heterosexual community. Health-care workers are at increased risk for exposure to HIV from needle-stick injuries and contamination with splashed or splattered body fluids. To assess the severity of exposure to HIV, several factors must be considered. These factors include the viral load of the patient; the nature of the fluid contacted; the type and severity of the exposure (needle-stick, mucous membrane; intact skin, broken skin); and the volume of contaminated body fluid.

CDC CLASSIFICATION OF AIDS

In 1993, the Centers for Disease Control and Prevention revised its diagnostic guidelines for AIDS. The document, entitled "1993 Revised Classification System for HIV Infection and Expanded Surveillance" (CDC), is a case definition for AIDS based on clinical conditions associated with HIV. The report identifies three categories of AIDS.

Category A

The first category consists of the following criteria:

> Asymptomatic HIV infection
> Persistent general enlargement of the lymph nodes
> Acute HIV infection with illness or a history of HIV infection

Category B

The second category of AIDS includes the above plus symptomatic conditions such as:

> Oral or vaginal candidiasis
> Fever or diarrhea for longer than one month
> At least two distinct episodes of shingles
> Pelvic inflammatory disease
> Peripheral neuropathy

There are other conditions associated with category B; however, EMS professionals rarely come across these cases.

Category C

The third classification is category C, which includes conditions not seen in the above two categories such as:

> Candidiasis of the airways, lungs, or esophagus
> Invasive cervical cancer
> Cryptosporidosis
> Cytomegalovirus
> Encephalopathy
> Herpes simplex infection with ulcers for more than one month
> Kaposi's sarcoma
> Wasting syndrome
> Other conditions EMS professionals rarely see

These guidelines developed by the CDC are currently in use; however, revisions to the guidelines have been suggested and put into place to assess disease severity. Researchers in Virginia have implemented an illness staging scale and are studying its effectiveness on rating the disease although this scale is not in widespread use.

SIGNS AND SYMPTOMS

There are several signs and symptoms associated with HIV infection and, ultimately, AIDS.

These signs and symptoms of HIV infection and AIDS include:

Lymphadenopathy—generalized enlargement of the lymph nodes

Persistent low-grade (less than 101°F) fever

Night sweats where the patient awakens in a profuse perspiration

Anorexia

Nausea

Persistent diarrhea

Headache

Sore throat, perhaps accompanied by oral candidiasis

Kaposi's sarcoma

Fatigue

Weight loss

Muscle and joint aches and pains

Rash

Pneumonia, which can be accompanied by severe dyspnea

OPPORTUNISTIC INFECTIONS

As was mentioned earlier, HIV infection impairs the body's immune system, thus allowing infectious agents and other diseases to invade and infect with little or no opposition. There are a number of opportunistic infections that EMS professionals may see in AIDS patients. Although none of these signs or symptoms is diagnostic of HIV infection or AIDS, they are all associated with the disease and its progression, especially with opportunistic infections.

Some opportunistic infections seen in the field are *Pneumocystis carinii* pneumonia, Kaposi's sarcoma, toxoplasmosis, cytomegalovirus, *cryptosporidium enterocolitis,* and *Candida albicans.* Below is a brief description of each condition.

Pneumocystis Carinii Pneumonia

This is pneumonia caused by what some researchers call a protozoa and others call a fungus. It leads to severe dyspnea, fever, productive cough, and cyanosis. The sputum contains plasma cells and other lung debris and, if untreated, can lead to severe hypoxia and death.

Kaposi's Sarcoma

Kaposi's sarcoma is a malignant tumor that appears blue-red in color. Typically, it appears on the lower extremities but can spread to other parts of the body, including internal organs.

Toxoplasmosis

Also called cat scratch fever, toxoplasmosis is caused by infection by the protozoa *Toxoplasma gondii.* The invading protozoa causes the development of cysts in tissues including the heart, lungs, liver, skin, muscles, and brain.

Cytomegalovirus

A member of the herpes family of viruses, it causes fever and inflammation of the liver and lungs. In AIDS patients, cytomegalovirus can also affect the central nervous system and kidneys along with ulcerations of the large intestines and esophagus.

Cryptosporidium Enterocolitis

Cryptosporidium is another protozoa that commonly thrives in the intestines of many different animals. When it invades humans, especially immunocompromised patients, the infection causes severe diarrhea accompanied by weight loss. Other signs and symptoms associated with cryptosporidium infection include fever and abdominal pain.

Candida Albicans

Candidiasis is caused by a yeast-like fungus that is commonly and normally found in the mouth, skin, intestines, and vagina. *Candida albicans* is the usual culprit in vaginal yeast infections and cases of oral thrush. In AIDS patients, severe cases of oral candidiasis can enter into the throat and esophagus causing difficult or painful swallowing. Lesions in the mouth appear as white patches over an inflamed area. Infection of the airways by *Candida albicans* can cause chest pain along with difficult breathing.

PERSONAL PROTECTION

The best protection against infection with HIV is using universal precautions. Wear gloves when examining any patient where blood is present or suspected, or when exposure to blood during the patient's treatment is expected. Wear mask, goggles, and gown whenever splashing or spattering of blood is likely.

According to the CDC's *HIV/AIDS Surveillance Report* issued in December 1998, a total of 188 health-care workers have contracted AIDS or HIV. Of that total, only 54 have documented occupational transmission of the virus whereas 134 have a possible occupational transmission of HIV. In the data, 12 EMTs and paramedics have experienced a possible occupational transmission of HIV, yet no documented transmission of HIV has occurred in EMS personnel. Although the incidence of seroconversion is low among EMTs and paramedics, it is extremely important to use precautions when caring for a patient who is, or may be, HIV positive.

After contact with the patient, be sure to dispose of contaminated waste properly and clean the patient compartment and any exposed equipment thoroughly with an approved disinfectant. After cleaning the vehicle, hands should be washed with a disinfectant soap.

There is no cure or vaccine against HIV at this time. Controlled studies are underway to test a vaccine, but widespread use may be years away. With the recent discovery of the origin of HIV, researchers can focus on finding a cure for the disease and a vaccination against infection. Recent studies have shown that the drug cocktails currently being used are reducing the viral load in infected patients. Occasionally, after using these drugs, some patients have shown no evidence of the virus in the blood. Researchers warn, however, that there could be hidden reservoirs of virus waiting to be released if the drugs are withdrawn.

A word of caution is appropriate here. There is evidence that variations of HIV are being transmitted within the United States that are resistant to the currently available drug therapy. It is estimated that up to 30 percent of the newly infected patients have a variation of HIV that does not respond to one of the 13 drugs used to treat HIV-positive and AIDS patients. It is important to follow your agency's Infection Control Program to protect against accidental exposure.

If an EMT or paramedic is exposed to HIV, he or she should follow the agency's postexposure control program, which includes testing and counseling as well as other options. In Chapter 9, Putting It All Together, we provide additional information about an Infection Control Program. There are currently no FDA-approved HIV test kits that give the results of the test at home. Test kits can be used at home to obtain a blood sample to send to an approved laboratory for testing. Results are kept confidential. A recent development is the advent of a rapid HIV test that is available in a clinic setting. The test, assessing for HIV antibodies, can provide results in 25 to 35 minutes. There are false positives and false negatives so, should the results show positive, the more thorough Western blot test is conducted. Negative tests should be repeated at a future date.

Some studies advocate the use of what is called Post Exposure Prophylaxis (PEP). This therapy includes the use of antiretroviral drugs currently used to treat HIV. Although the PEP program is not 100 percent effective, it has been shown to be beneficial.

☎ YOU MAKE THE CALL

You respond to an apartment complex where you are greeted by a concerned family telling you that someone at home is very ill. They are somewhat vague about the nature of the problem until you get inside the apartment. You are taken to a 29-year-old man who is laying on a couch in the living room. He is dressed only in shorts and you notice that he is diaphoretic and febrile to the touch. He tells you that he is having trouble breathing and swallowing. Listening to breath sounds reveals bilateral congestion with decreased breath sounds in the lung bases. The patient opens his mouth to show you several white patches on a reddened surface. The patches appear to extend into the patient's throat. At the same time you are assessing the patient, a family member approaches and tells you the man has recently been diagnosed with AIDS.

What are the signs and symptoms of AIDS?

What are the possible causes for the man's difficulty breathing?

What is the most likely cause for the man's difficult swallowing?

In caring for this man, what personal protective equipment would you use?

SUMMARY

HIV and AIDS are devastating. Once infected with HIV, the patient's life is significantly shortened. This chapter has briefly covered HIV and AIDS, discussing the signs, symptoms, and nature of the disease. Because the virus depends upon the host to copy itself, the virus attaches to T-helper lymphocytes and uses their genes to replicate. By using the host cell's genes, the cell dies. The end result is the body's inability to ward off opportunistic infections. Patients with HIV will ultimately develop AIDS and succumb to the disease.

This chapter also talked about the signs and symptoms of AIDS as they pertain to the guidelines published by the CDC. It also discussed the opportunistic infections that can overwhelm a weakened immune system and cause the patient's death.

Personal protection is key to preventing HIV exposure. Wearing personal protective equipment and disinfecting the vehicle and its equipment thoroughly is essential. By using the proper precautions, risk of infection can be minimized.

8

With a Jaundiced Eye
Hepatitis—An Alphabet Soup

OBJECTIVES

At the end of the chapter, the reader will be able to:

1. Define the following terms:

Co-infection	Enteric infection
Fulminating	Jaundice
Palpation	Parenteral infection

2. State the methods of transmitting hepatitis A, B, and C viruses.
3. Describe the three phases of hepatitis infection.
4. List three signs or symptoms commonly found in hepatitis infections.
5. List the risk factors associated with contracting hepatitis C.

Although there is risk for exposure to a myriad of infectious diseases, a few diseases have higher risk for EMTs and paramedics. Two of these diseases—hepatitis and HIV—are bloodborne pathogens as well as sexually transmitted diseases. They can easily be transmitted to EMS personnel if precautions are not taken.

Hepatitis has been gaining attention in the medical and trade journals as well as other media since medical researchers have noticed an increasing prevalence of hepatitis C. Because of the varieties and the risks for EMS professionals associated with hepatitis, this entire chapter is devoted to this potentially fatal viral disease.

WORDS TO KNOW

Asymptomatic   Having no signs or symptoms of disease.

Cirrhosis   A degenerative condition of the liver in which the lobes of the liver are covered with fibrous tissue and the liver tissue is infiltrated with fat. Liver function deteriorates.

Co-infection   A secondary infection with another virus or bacteria.

Enteric infection   An infection occurring in the small intestine.

Fulminating   Occurring suddenly and with great intensity.

Hepatitis   Inflammation of the liver.

Icteric phase   Phase of hepatitis characterized by jaundice.

Jaundice   Symptom of hepatitis characterized by the yellowing of the skin and white portions of the eyes.

Oral-fecal contamination   Contamination of food, clothing, or other item by fecal matter that is then transferred to the mouth.

Palpation   Examination by touching.

Parenteral infection   Infection that occurs by subcutaneous, intramuscular, or intravenous injection.

Prodromal phase   Symptoms indicating the onset of an illness.

NATURE AND SPREAD OF THE DISEASE

Hepatitis is a viral disease that, in its simplest definition, means inflammation of the liver. Early in the twentieth century, two varieties of the disease were identified. One type was spread in the intestines by ingestion of contaminated food or water (enteric infection). The other type was spread by contact with blood or other body fluids (parenteral infection). With further research and increased information, different viruses were identified as causing hepatitis.

Currently, there are several viruses associated with hepatitis that result in swelling and enlargement of the liver along with mild to severe liver damage. Some forms of hepatitis have been associated with chronic liver disease leading to liver failure or liver cancer. The different viruses have been labeled A, B, C, D, E, F, and G.

Hepatitis A

Hepatitis A, formerly called *infectious hepatitis*, is an enteric infection causing between 125,000 to 200,000 cases in the United States each year. Over the past several years, the number of reported cases has been increasing. Of these infections, a small number will die from a severe, fulminating case of the disease. It is estimated that 33 percent of all Americans will show evidence of past infection by hepatitis A virus (HAV).

Spread of the disease is most commonly by oral-fecal contamination. Although this sounds somewhat ominous, oral-fecal contamination can occur in several different ways. A common method of transmission is exposure to contaminated water. If sewage spills into a body of water, people in contact with that water can become infected. Another example of transmission is by eating contaminated shellfish. Shellfish such as clams living in water contaminated by raw sewage will become infectious agents and transmit HAV to anyone who eats the raw clams. Another example is contamination from one person to another, especially if the infectious person fails to wash or inadequately washes his or her hands after using the bathroom. Contamination by soiled eating utensils is also possible. Finally, sexual contact with an infectious person can transmit HAV.

Hepatitis B

Hepatitis B, a parenteral infection, formerly called *serum hepatitis*, is expected to infect between 140,000 and 320,000 Americans annually. Infection with the hepatitis B virus (HBV) is associated with a higher complication rate and typically causes just under 20,000 hospital admissions each year with 140 to 320 deaths. Of all HBV cases, up to 10 percent will develop chronic infections. An estimated 5,000 to 6,000 people will die each year from chronic liver disease—including liver cancer caused by HBV. The incidence of HBV infections declined between 1985 and 1993 due to an HBV vaccination program; however, there has been a recent increase in the number of reported cases, especially among high-risk categories.

HBV is transmitted by contact with an infected person's blood or body fluids. Sexual contact with an infectious person can result in contracting hepatitis B. Those at particular risk for infection include IV drug abusers, sexually active men and women in contact with infected people, health-care workers (including EMS personnel), and patients on hemodialysis. Unlike the HIV, the hepatitis B virus is able to survive for long periods of time outside the human body.

Hepatitis C

Hepatitis C, also a parenteral infection, has been called parenteral non-A, non-B hepatitis and is estimated to infect from 28,000 to 180,000 Americans each year. Current estimates show that 4 million people in the United States are infected with the hepatitis C virus (HCV) with only a fourth of those knowing they are infected. Other estimates indicate that over 170 million people worldwide are infected with HCV. Over the past two decades, the occurrence of new cases stabilized and had gradually declined. Recent research indicates the incidence of new cases to be increasing, especially among those at high risk for the disease.

HCV infection is associated with a high incidence of chronic infection (over 85 percent). Chronic infection results in chronic liver disease in 70 percent of infected people and is causing up to 10,000 deaths per year. The medical literature suggests that, over the next 10 years, the need for liver transplantation will increase 500 percent.

HCV is transmitted by bloodborne contamination or sexual contact. Whereas it was thought that HCV did not survive outside the body for any length of time, current evidence has shown that HCV can survive in dried blood for up to three weeks at normal room temperature.

People at risk for contracting HCV include IV drug abusers, patients on hemodialysis, health-care workers, individuals having sexual contact with those with HCV or people with multiple sexual contacts, and people who received blood or blood clotting factors prior to 1992. EMS professionals are at particular risk for exposure to HCV from needle-stick injuries or contact with a patient's blood, even dried blood that may be left on improperly cleaned equipment used on a prior patient. Exposure to HCV can be subtle and infection can be undetected. There are concerns among health-care professionals that HCV can even be spread by contact with contaminated personal items such as a toothbrush or a razor.

Hepatitis D

Another distinct virus causing inflammation of the liver is the hepatitis D virus (HDV), also called *delta hepatitis.* HDV is associated with a simultaneous infection or co-infection with HBV. The nature of the virus requires an association with another virus because it cannot replicate itself in the absence of the other virus. It is transmitted in the same manner as hepatitis B—by bloodborne or sexual contact. Most often, patients with HDV have a history of IV drug abuse. A patient with HBV who suddenly deteriorates should be suspected of having a co-infection with HDV.

Hepatitis E

Hepatitis E has also been called enteric non-A, non-B hepatitis and is caused by infection with the hepatitis E virus (HEV). Although HEV has rarely been found in the United States, major outbreaks of hepatitis associated with HEV have been found in third world countries. With the ease of travel between the United States and developing nations, the spread of HEV is increasing.

HEV is typically seen in young to middle-aged patients. Pregnant women are most susceptible to severe disease. Women in their second to third trimester of pregnancy have a mortality rate approaching 20 percent with infection from HEV.

The disease is spread through exposure to contaminated food and water and by person-to-person contact especially after natural disasters with flooding or contamination of water sources by raw sewage.

Hepatitis F

There is controversy regarding the actual presence of another strain of hepatitis virus. In 1994, researchers in Europe isolated a virus not previously found that caused hepatitis. This non-A, non-B, non-C, non-E virus was found to cause inflammation of the liver when injected into study animals. Thus, the virus was named hepatitis F virus or HFV. Subsequent studies have failed to confirm the results of initial studies and HFV was dismissed as a separate infectious agent. According to the literature, there is no HFV.

Hepatitis G

Very little is known about the hepatitis G virus (HGV). However, a separate virus has been isolated from a small number of patients with acute hepatitis. It is estimated that from 900 to 2,000 cases of hepatitis G occur annually in the United States.

From the information available thus far, HGV is a bloodborne disease, transmitted by way of transfusion and IV drug abuse. It is often found as a co-infection with HCV.

SIGNS AND SYMPTOMS

There are three phases of hepatitis—the prodromal phase, the icteric phase, and the recovery phase. The signs and symptoms of the various infections are fairly similar. At times, the signs and symptoms are so mild that the patient does not realize he or she may be ill with hepatitis. With other infections, the patient may be asymptomatic.

In the initial or prodromal phase of hepatitis, the patient will complain of flu-like symptoms including fatigue, weakness, loss of appetite, nausea, and vomiting. Frequently, a fever will also be present. One characteristic early symptom in smokers is the distaste for cigarettes. As the disease progresses, hives develop, causing the patient to itch. Although this is more prevalent in hepatitis B, recent evidence suggests that severe itching of the skin may be the initial finding in HCV infection. This may be especially true in patients with chronic hepatitis C. Approximately three to ten days later, the patient's urine will turn dark brown. The patient's liver may also be enlarged and tender on abdominal palpation.

Jaundice appears in what is called the icteric phase. The initial signs of jaundice appear in the eyes, when the sclera, or whites, of the eyes turns yellow. In hepatitis A, the eyes might show the only evidence of jaundice. In other cases of hepatitis, jaundice spreads over the entire body. The yellow discoloration of the skin will peak in one to two weeks, then gradually fade during what is known as the recovery phase.

Hepatitis usually resolves in four to eight weeks. Hepatitis A rarely develops into a chronic infection; however, hepatitis B and C have a high incidence of becoming chronic. Chronic hepatitis can cause a mild, persistent inflammation of the liver. Chronic active hepatitis can result in liver damage such as cirrhosis, liver cancer, and liver failure. Hepatitis carries a high percentage of chronic infection that will, according to some researchers, result in a significant increase in the number of liver transplants in the future. Patients at risk for chronic hepatitis will be notified of their increased chance of infection and be asked to be tested for HCV.

PERSONAL PROTECTION

All health-care workers are at risk for infection by any of the hepatitis viruses. In EMS, as in other allied health professions, workers are at particular risk for exposure to hepatitis A, B, and C viruses.

Hepatitis A and E

As was mentioned earlier, hepatitis A and E are considered enteric infections—with exposure by fecal or oral-fecal contamination. A patient with HAV can transmit the virus by items contaminated by his or her feces. Even an occult contamination could pose a substantial risk. In areas of poor sanitation, particularly in an area affected by a natural disaster, when contamination of drinking water is increased, there may be substantial risk of fecal contamination. Hands should be thoroughly washed after every patient contact, and disinfect or decontaminate any equipment that may have been in contact with an infected patient.

Presently a vaccine against HAV is available and has been shown to be highly effective against the disease. If you have not received the HAV vaccination and the risk for exposure to the virus is high, immune globulin (gamma globulin) can be administered both pre- and postexposure, protecting from infection by HAV or HEV.

Hepatitis B

Since the development of a hepatitis B vaccine, the number of cases of hepatitis B has been decreasing. However, the incidence of HBV infection has increased in certain high-risk groups—sexually active heterosexuals, homosexual men, and IV drug abusers. Because the disease is a bloodborne pathogen, contamination by an infected patient's blood poses a significant risk for unvaccinated EMS personnel. Regardless of prior vaccination, universal precautions should be used to reduce potential exposure to a patient's blood. Gloves are essential and, if blood splatter is likely, a face mask, goggles, and gown are also indicated. Proper hand washing and equipment decontamination is critical.

Recently, the media have reported an alleged association of HBV vaccination with severe adverse reactions including multiple sclerosis, chronic fatigue syndrome, rheumatoid arthritis, optic neuritis, or other autoimmune disorders. According to the Centers for Disease Control and Prevention, there is no confirmation of any association between HBV vaccination and any of these conditions. The Centers for Disease Control and Prevention strongly urges continuation of the vaccination program to prevent hepatitis B.

Hepatitis C

Hepatitis C has been labeled a silent epidemic. Because there is no vaccine to protect against HCV, proper screening is the first means of reducing risk. A blood test can determine HCV exposure. However, the test may not be needed unless several risk factors are met. These factors include:

- Exposure to infected blood
- Sharing personal grooming items (toothbrush, razor) with infected person
- Chronic kidney dialysis.
- Organ transplantation prior to 1992
- Sexual relations with an infected individual
- Tattoo or manicure with equipment that may not have been disinfected
- Surgery or dental work with equipment that may not have been disinfected
- IV drug abuse or sharing needles with potentially infectious people

If any of the above risk factors have occurred, contact a physician about a blood test to detect antibodies for HCV. The Food and Drug Administration has recently approved an over-the-counter blood collecting kit that can be used at home to obtain a blood sample that then is mailed to a laboratory for analysis.

☎ YOU MAKE THE CALL

The patient you have been called to see is a 57-year-old man complaining of severe right upper quadrant abdominal pain. He states that every inch of his skin is extremely tender to the touch. You note the man's skin is jaundiced as are the sclera (whites) of his eyes. You also find minor bleeding from a wound on the man's right leg sustained when he became dizzy and fell. The man's wife tells you he contracted hepatitis C many months ago and had been on interferon therapy for the past year.

In preparing to care for this man, what universal precautions should you use in patient assessment as well as in dressing and bandaging the injury?

After the call has been completed, you note some dried blood on a cabinet. Is this dried blood a source for transmitting hepatitis C? How would you disinfect the cabinet?

There is no cure for HCV. A few therapies have been developed and show promise. These treatments include alpha interferon and ribavirin. However, neither treatment alone or in combination with other medication has been totally effective in curing the disease. A recent study has shown that when used in combination, only 38 percent of those treated with alpha interferon and ribavirin responded favorably.

Proper precautions with all patients are important. Wear gloves at all times when in contact with a patient, and when blood spattering is possible, use a face mask, goggles, and gown. Because the virus can survive for a prolonged period of time in dried blood, all equipment in contact with or exposed to the patient's blood must be thoroughly cleaned and disinfected. Uniforms with blood spatters must be removed and laundered appropriately. Soiled clothing, including shoes, should not be taken home.

SUMMARY

This chapter has been devoted to a single infectious disease—hepatitis. The severity of the illness and the risks that EMS professionals face require that special attention be given to this illness.

Hepatitis, or the inflammation of the liver, can be caused by any of several viruses. They can enter the body by way of the gastrointestinal system, the skin, or other parenteral port of entry. Once inside the body, the hepatitis viruses have the potential to destroy the liver with an acute or, in the case of HBV or HCV, chronic infection.

Whereas there is a prevention for hepatitis B—the hepatitis vaccine—there is no cure for hepatitis C. Two drugs currently being used, alpha interferon and ribavirin, offer some hope to overcome the infection.

Proper protection including the use of gloves, masks, goggles, and gowns reduces the possibility of infection with HBV and HCV. Proper disposal of sharps and the cleaning of contaminated equipment reduce the risk of exposure.

Putting It All Together
Infection Control Program

OBJECTIVES

At the end of the chapter, the reader will be able to:

1. Given a list of governmental agencies; be able to identify OSHA as the agency responsible for the Bloodborne Pathogens Standard.
2. List the components of the Bloodborne Pathogens Standard.
3. State the role of the Infection Control Officer.
4. State the appropriate procedure for handling clothing that has been contaminated with blood including procedures for removing clothing from the employee.
5. Correctly identify the personal protective equipment to be worn when in contact with the patient.
6. List the situations that require the use of a respirator.
7. List the components of the training program required by OSHA for all EMS personnel.
8. State the instances when an employee can decline vaccination for hepatitis B.

In the early and mid-1980s, EMS organizations began realizing the importance of taking precautions against bloodborne and airborne diseases. With mounting pressure from labor, the federal Occupational Safety and Health Administration (OSHA) developed its first workplace safety standard. Originally intended for employers to provide health-care workers a safe environment, the standard has since been modified to include employee responsibility for protection against infection in the workplace. The Bloodborne Pathogens Standard implemented in 1991 requires employers and employees to contribute to a safe work environment.

WORDS TO KNOW

Engineering controls Methods used in the workplace that reduce or eliminate risk of exposure to an infectious agent such as hazardous waste disposal system.

HEPA mask High Efficiency Particulate Air mask is a type of respirator.

High level disinfection Disinfecting surfaces with an agent designed to destroy most bacteria and viruses including TB. Bacterial spores may not be destroyed.

Intermediate level disinfection Using a disinfectant to clean surfaces which will destroy viruses and bacteria including TB, but will not kill bacterial spores.

Low level disinfection Using disinfectants to clean surfaces which will destroy some viruses, but bacterial spores and TB will not be killed.

Personal protective equipment Equipment issued to the employee to be used while caring for a patient to reduce the risk of exposure to an infectious agent.

Postexposure procedures A part of the Infection Control Plan that details the steps taken after an employee has been exposed to an infectious agent.

Respirator A special mask designed to filter dust particles that may be carrying the TB bacteria.

Sterilization Disinfecting by destroying all microorganisms.

Universal precautions An approach to infection control by considering that all body fluids are potentially infectious.

Workplace practice controls The employees' role in reducing risk of exposure including washing of hands and properly disposing of sharps.

OSHA is constantly developing standards and guidelines to ensure workplace safety. For example, with an increased risk of exposure to tuberculosis, especially drug-resistant strains of the bacteria, OSHA is developing guidelines for prevention of the transmission of tuberculosis. Coupled with tuberculosis prevention guidelines from the Centers for Disease Control and Prevention, we have seen a concerted effort among all health-care workers to reduce the risk of exposure to these deadly diseases.

OSHA's Bloodborne Pathogens Standard, along with the CDC's guidelines for controlling the transmission of tuberculosis, requires each employer to establish an Infection Control Plan available to all employees. This plan consists of several components, which include:

- Identifying employees at risk for exposure
- Developing an exposure control plan and schedule for implementing it
- Creating a plan that establishes postexposure procedures

EXPOSURE CONTROL PLAN

In creating an exposure control plan, both the CDC and OSHA have made recommendations to prevent or reduce exposure to tuberculosis and bloodborne pathogens. These recommendations include:

- Universal precautions
- Engineering controls
- Workplace practice controls
- Personal protective equipment
- Training programs
- Vaccinations against hepatitis B
- Labeling and handling infectious waste
- Postexposure procedures

In order to enforce the CDC's and OSHA's guidelines, someone within the EMS agency must be responsible for the Infection Control Program. A sample Infection Control Program can be found in the Appendix of this book. Often, a designated Infection Control Officer oversees all agency policies and procedures concerning bloodborne pathogens. The Infection Control Officer monitors the employer and employees' compliance with federal, state, and local rules or regulations. The Infection Control Officer also monitors the bloodborne pathogen training program and assures that everyone has been issued appropriate personal protective equipment.

Although the employer has a large responsibility in ensuring a safe work environment, employees also share in that responsibility. This includes following and using universal precautions along with personal protective equipment. Everyone must adhere to workplace practice controls.

UNIVERSAL PRECAUTIONS

According to the Standard, universal precautions are "an approach to infection control." Under the concept of bloodborne pathogens, consider that all body fluids, especially those containing blood, are potentially infectious. If the nature of the fluid is undetermined, consider it hazardous and a potential risk for transmission of HIV, HBV, HCV, and other infectious agents.

ENGINEERING CONTROLS

Engineering controls include ways to reduce or eliminate exposure to an infectious agent. For example, employers are to ensure adequate hand washing facilities on the premises or, when hand washing facilities are not available, to provide an antiseptic hand cleaner and cloth or paper towels (see photo). Antiseptic towelettes can be substituted for the waterless hand cleanser and paper towels (see photo that follows).

Another engineering control consists of providing equipment designed to reduce the risk of exposure to blood or other body fluids. For example, an

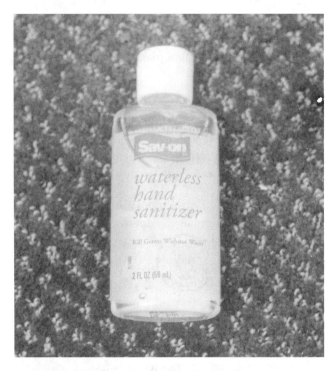

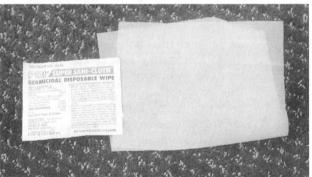

Waterless hand cleaners can be used until soap and water are available.

appropriately labeled sharps container should be easily accessible for disposing contaminated needles and syringes. Another type of safety equipment are the sheathed suction catheters, which, after insertion into the patient's airway, are withdrawn into a plastic sheath to reduce spatter or splashing of secretions. Syringes with needles that retract into the syringe or have a protective sheath have been introduced to EMS providers (see photo that follows). These items prevent accidental exposure to contaminated needles by retracting the needle into the syringe or allowing the sharp to be surrounded by a plastic covering.

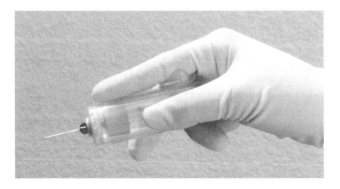

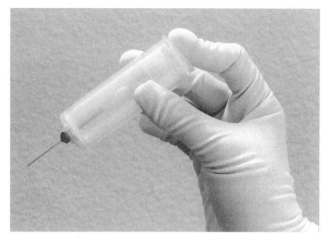

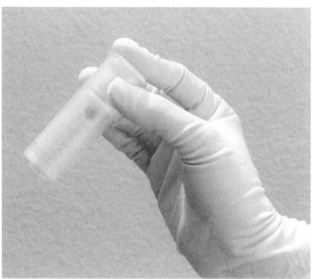

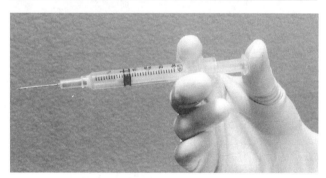

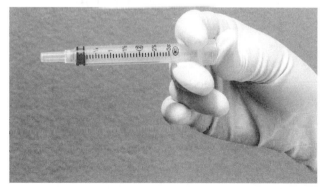

VanishPoint™ blood collection holder and syringe from Retractable Technologies.

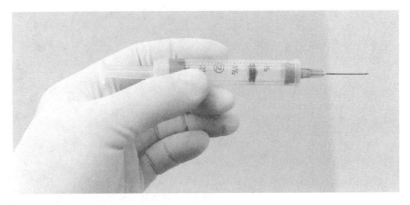

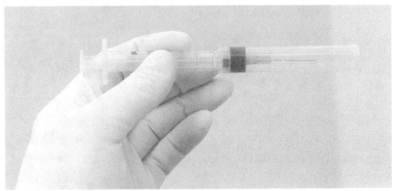

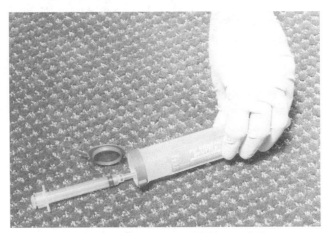

Safety-Lok™ from Becton Dickinson & Co.

At times, it might be necessary to place the sharp into a portable container for safekeeping until it can be disposed of properly. There are a few transportable containers such as the Sharps Shuttle™ and the Protex Sharpseal™. Once used, sharps can be scooped into the Sharp Shuttle or inserted into the Sharpseal to prevent accidental needle-stick injuries. See the following photos illustrating these two containers.

The employer must also provide cleaning supplies and equipment such as disinfectant solutions and trash containers labeled for the disposal of hazardous waste (see photo on page 103). For cleaning or disinfecting contaminated equipment at the station, the employer must also provide a safe place to clean the equipment. Hoses, cleaning supplies, and appropriate drainage of contaminated water must be available.

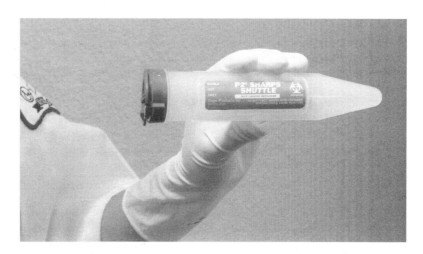

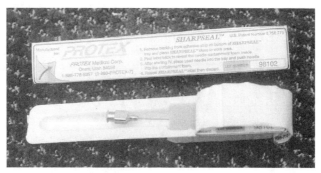

Transportable containers – Sharps Shuttle™ and Sharpseal™.

WORKPLACE PRACTICE CONTROLS

Whereas the employer must provide a safe environment, employees have the responsibility for safe workplace practices. OSHA's guidelines suggest several practices that can be used to reduce risk.

Eating, drinking, smoking, applying cosmetics, or using any personal items that may come into contact with infectious waste must be avoided. Many employers have rules that strictly prohibit eating, drinking, or smoking inside the ambulance cab. "Why would this be a problem after or in between calls?" The answer is simple. Consider this scenario:

You and your partner respond to a motor vehicle accident and provide care for a seriously injured patient. You have followed infection control guidelines and used gloves, face mask, and eye protection to avoid risk of exposure to the patient's blood or body fluids. After caring for the patient on the scene, you load the patient into the ambulance and secure the gurney for transportation. Your partner will be driving to the emergency department. After closing the rear doors, your partner opens the driver's door of the ambulance, climbs into the cab, puts the ambulance into gear, and heads to the hospital. As you depart the scene, your partner picks up the radio microphone and notifies dispatch of your status. So far, everything is proceeding smoothly! Or is it? Did your partner remove his or her gloves before closing the patient compartment doors or climbing into the cab of the ambulance? If not, think of all the surfaces he or she has contaminated with the patient's body fluids. Then, ask yourself, is it safe to consume food inside that cab?

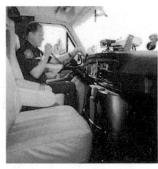

List all surfaces in the cab that could be contaminated by careless infection control.

To prevent contamination of the cab, the driver should remove his or her gloves prior to entering the cab. Additionally, the hands should be cleaned with a waterless solution or disinfectant towelette. However, this is not always feasible. To reduce any delay in transporting the patient, the driver can double-glove upon arrival at the scene. By wearing two gloves on each hand, the driver simply removes the contaminated pair and leaves them in the back of the ambulance prior to driving to the hospital.

Bending or recapping contaminated needles is not permitted. Dispose of all sharps in an approved container. If you must recap any needle, do not use a two-handed method. There are at least three different ways to recap a contaminated needle. First, place the cap on a flat surface then scoop the cap with the needle. Do not attempt this in a moving vehicle.

Forceps or hemostats can be used to hold the cap while inserting the contaminated needle. This method is also unsafe for use in a moving vehicle.

A third method for recapping a contaminated needle is to secure the cap under the sole of your shoe and insert the needle into the cap. If you miss the cap, you might stab the sole of your shoe. You can use this technique in a moving vehicle.

At no time should the seat cushion be used as a temporary needle holder until the sharp can be placed into an approved container. Keep in mind that the hepatitis C virus can survive up to three weeks in dried blood. This practice has been seen in a few EMS agencies in the past and, with the availability of appropriate equipment, should have been discontinued.

Be sure to wash hands immediately after removing the gloves. Wash hands thoroughly using soap and water (see photos that follow). Be sure to scrub under the fingernails as well as around the wrists and approximately 2 to 3 inches up the forearm. Washing hands and wrists should be for a minimum of 10 seconds and, if possible, take at least 3 minutes. Simply rinsing hands under tap water is insufficient. If no water is available, use the water-

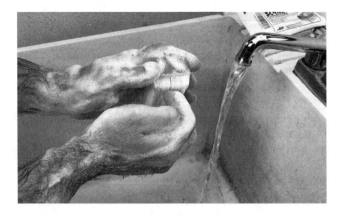

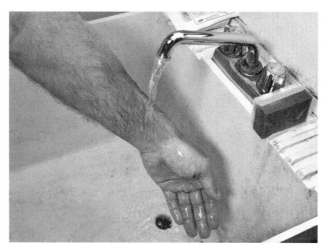
Thoroughly wash hands with soap and water.

less antiseptic solution or antiseptic towelette. However, when soap and water become available, you are required to wash your hands thoroughly.

On a particularly messy call there might be blood or body fluids on your shoes. Be sure to clean them thoroughly with disinfectant solution. Scrub around the soles of the shoes, paying particular attention to where the sole is attached to the top of the shoe.

If your uniform has been soiled with blood or body fluids, remove the clothing in a way that prevents exposure of the contaminated clothing to your mucous membranes. If necessary, cut off contaminated clothing and dispose of it properly. Because there is a chance of soiling the uniform, have a spare uniform or change of clothes at work.

The employer is to provide laundry facilities for cleaning contaminated clothing. Do not take contaminated clothing home. Family or friends could be exposed to the patients that you examined and treated. Change clothing before leaving the workplace.

Disinfecting the equipment and vehicle is critical. As has been mentioned before, the hepatitis C virus can survive in dried blood for up to three weeks. Thus, it is critical to clean thoroughly all equipment and surfaces that may have come in contact with the patient's blood or body fluids.

Once the patient has been turned over to emergency department staff, it is important that all contaminated items be cleaned or disposed of according to federal, state, and local laws as well as the agency's infection control procedures. Make sure infectious waste is placed in approved, leak-proof containers and disinfect reusable items. Keep in mind there is a distinct difference between cleaning and disinfecting. Cleaning refers to removing dirt and debris usually with water and occasionally with a cleaning agent such as soap. It does not remove or destroy bacteria or viruses. Disinfecting refers to the destruction of bacteria, viruses, and fungi. Disinfecting an item does not destroy bacterial spores. A soiled item must first be cleaned with soap and water because some disinfectants cannot penetrate blood, pus, or other organic substances.

When disinfecting equipment, wear appropriate personal protective equipment based on how materials will be decontaminated. If using a disinfectant to spray on a surface and then wipe off, gloves, mask, and protective eyewear will probably suffice. If disinfecting a larger area using mops, hoses, or large quantities of disinfectant, boots and a water-repellant gown in addition to the other personal protective equipment may be needed. For heavily soiled items, clean first with soap and water, then carry out the disinfecting procedures that follow.

To disinfect or decontaminate exposed items, use one or more of four different methods. Depending on the nature of contamination, use a low-, intermediate-, or high-level disinfection process or have the equipment sterilized.

Low-level disinfection uses Environmental Protection Agency (EPA) registered disinfectants such as Lysol® to destroy many bacteria and fungi. Some viruses will be destroyed; however, these disinfectants will not kill bacterial spores or the tuberculosis bacteria. You can use these disinfectants to remove body fluids, but you should not rely upon them to destroy any remaining bacteria or viruses.

Intermediate-level disinfection uses an EPA-registered germicide and destroys viruses, fungi, and bacteria, including tuberculosis bacteria. However, it does not destroy bacterial spores. You can use a 1:10 to 1:100 bleach in water solution to achieve intermediate-level disinfection. Care should be taken when exposing equipment made of fabric to any bleach solution. Alcohol, such as isopropyl alcohol or rubbing alcohol, can be used, but using it requires at least five minutes of "wet" contact. Alcohol-containing solutions can also damage some fabric or rubber materials.

High-level disinfection using products such as Cidex Plus® or a similar disinfectant will destroy most infectious agents except some bacterial spores. Use this solution to disinfect reusable equipment such as forceps, laryngoscope handles, and blades. Reusable suction equipment that has been contaminated should also be decontaminated with a high-level disinfectant.

Sterilization is rarely needed for equipment used in the prehospital setting. Sterilizing equipment destroys all organisms. Sterilization of equipment can be achieved by exposing the item to steam, gas, or radiation. Occasionally, you can sterilize an instrument by soaking it in a disinfecting solution for a period of six to ten hours depending on the manufacturer's recommendations.

PERSONAL PROTECTIVE EQUIPMENT

The employer must provide equipment that helps reduce the risk of exposure. Although this equipment is to be provided at no cost to the employee, it is up to the employee to wear it. Examples of personal protective equipment include gloves, masks, face shields, goggles, respirators, gowns, and shoe covers. In some situations, personal protective equipment may also include CPR barriers and resuscitation devices. In rare circumstances, when donning protective equipment will delay health care, the EMT or paramedic can choose not to wear personal protective equipment for a brief period of time.

The personal protective equipment must be designed to prevent exposure under normal circumstances. This means that it should not permit infectious material to reach your clothing, undergarments, skin, or mucous membranes. See the following photo for examples of personal protective equipment.

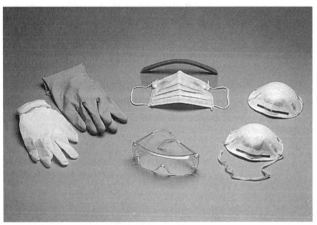

Personal Protective Equipment

Activity	Gloves	Eyewear	Mask	Gown
Uncontrolled bleeding	Y	Y	Y	Y
Controlled bleeding	Y	N	N	N
Childbirth	Y	Y	Y	Y
Endotracheal intubation	Y	Y	Y	N
Oral/nasal suctioning	Y	Y	Y	Y
Cleaning instruments	Y	Y	Y	Y
Taking blood pressure	N[*]	N	N	N
Giving an injection	Y	N	N	N
Taking a temperature	Y	N	N	N
Cleaning patient compartment	Y	N[**]	N[**]	N[**]

[*] If the patient's arm is contaminated with blood or body fluids, then wear gloves.

[**] If patient compartment is heavily contaminated with blood, then use eyewear, mask, and gown.

Workplace rules have been implemented that require the use of specific types of personal protective equipment while caring for patients with certain conditions or when specific risks are present. The CDC and National Fire Protection Association (NFPA) have developed standards for use of personal protective equipment. Although these standards are similar, there are some differences. The table above reflects the NFPA standards.

The above list only partially reflects the various situations encountered in the field. It would be impossible to cover every patient care scenario and identify which personal protective equipment should be used. In most cases, the EMS professional will have to rely upon his or her own judgment to determine which equipment will protect best. Whenever there is a risk of splashing or spattering of blood or body fluids, be sure to use eyewear, masks, and gown.

Gloves

The CDC, NFPA, OSHA, and other regulatory agencies require the use of latex or vinyl gloves whenever there is a possibility of exposure to blood or body fluids. In most patient care situations, disposable gloves are an effective barrier against exposure to bloodborne pathogens. According to the Bloodborne Pathogen Standard:

Gloves shall be worn when it can be reasonably anticipated that the employee may have hand contact with blood, other potentially infectious materials, mucous membranes, and non-intact skin; when performing vascular access procedures and when handling or touching contaminated items or surfaces.

Additionally, the Standard says that you will change gloves

as soon as practical when contaminated or as soon as feasible if they are torn, punctured, or when their ability to function as a barrier is compromised.

Some people are sensitive to latex and may develop an allergic reaction after wearing latex gloves for a prolonged time. People who are sensitive to latex should consider wearing a vinyl glove or one made of nitrile. If that is not possible, contact the Infection Control Officer, supervisor, or physician about what is available.

Disposable gloves will not protect from sharp objects. Handle any sharp with care. Further, latex or vinyl gloves will not endure stressful tasks such as cleaning equipment or the inside of the vehicle. Use a heavy-duty rubber glove for cleaning equipment or the patient compartment of the vehicle. At the scene of a motor vehicle accident where a victim has to be extricated, wear work gloves over latex gloves.

If a glove tears and no exposure or contamination has occurred, remove both gloves and replace them after washing your hands. When accidentally exposed to a potentially infectious agent, follow the agency's exposure control plan.

For additional protection against organisms that could come in contact with the hands, some manufacturers have developed an antimicrobial lotion to be rubbed on the hands prior to donning gloves (see photo that follows). This lotion is not to be used as a substitute for wearing gloves.

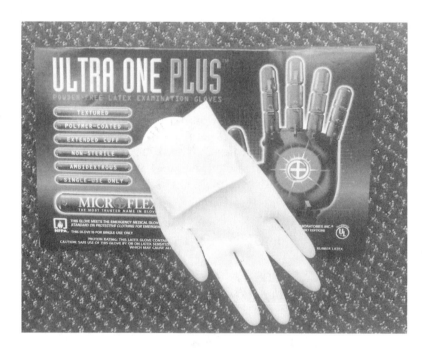

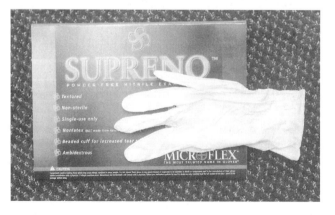

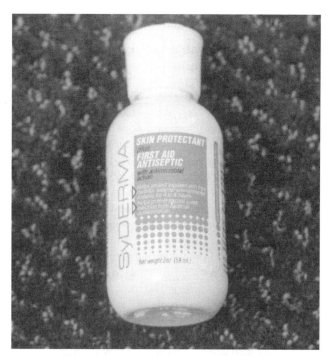

Skin protectant lotion can act as a barrier.

One portal of entry for infectious agents is through the mucous membranes of the eyes and nose. Use eye protection that will fit your face properly. If you wear glasses, use goggles that fit over eyeglasses (see photo that follows) or use side protectors to prevent blood from splashing into the eyes from the sides of the frames.

A protective face shield can be worn in place of goggles or protective glasses. Occasionally, it may serve as a substitute for a face mask. In the event of splashing or spattering of body fluids, the open bottom of the face shield may permit exposure to bloodborne pathogens.

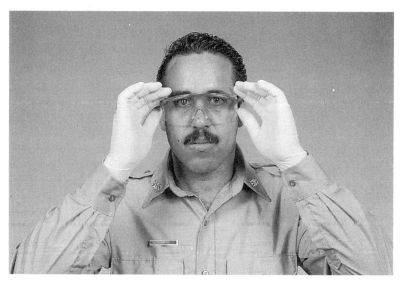

Properly fitting goggles protect the eyes from splashing.

In the event splashing or splattering of blood or body fluids is possible, you should wear a face mask to cover your mouth and nose. In most situations, a simple surgical face mask is sufficient. Most of the surgical masks used by EMS personnel are single-use paper-type masks secured to the head by elastic bands or ties. After securing the mask over the mouth and nose, a moldable metal band can be gently pinched to fit the mask properly around the nose. Occasionally, if wearing glasses, warm moist exhaled air causes the glasses to fog, obstructing vision. Should this happen, firmly pinch the band over the nose to seat the edges of the mask better. If glasses continue to become foggy, it might be necessary to place a small strip of adhesive tape over the upper edge of the face mask and secure the mask to the skin.

Some face masks combine the surgical face mask with protection for the eyes in the form of an eye shield. The combination mask and eye shield can be worn over regular glasses and eliminate the need for separate goggles.

The simple surgical face mask is not adequate to protect from airborne diseases, particularly tuberculosis. When called to care for a patient with tuberculosis, a special mask that filters out dust particles is needed. These masks, called High Efficiency Particulate Air (HEPA) masks or respirators, are effective at removing 95 to 99 percent of the dust particles that may be con-

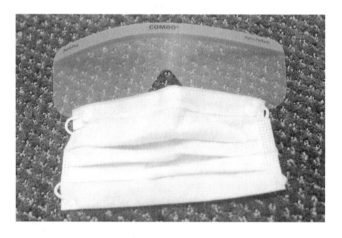

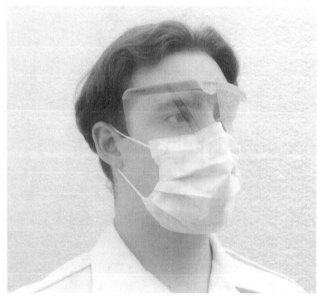

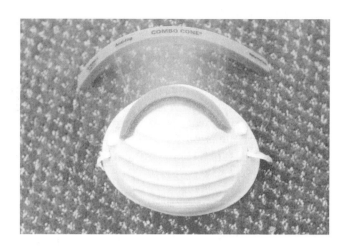

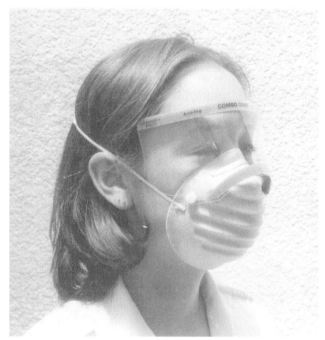

Combination face mask and eye shield.

taminated with *Mycobacterium tuberculosis.* Per current CDC recommendations, respirators must filter at least 95 percent of the dust particles. Prior CDC
guidelines indicated that the only acceptable respirator for use around patients with tuberculosis was the HEPA respirator. More recently, however,
nine classes of respirators meet CDC criteria.

It is imperative that the respirator fits properly and does not permit air to
leak around the edges of the device. If, after placing the respirator over the
mouth and nose, an air leak is detected, adjust the edges of the device to seal
the leak. After assuring proper fit of the respirator, store it properly by following these guidelines:

- Write your name on your respirator.
- Place your respirator in a paper bag. A plastic bag should not be used
  because the respirator may be moist. A damp respirator allows the growth
  of bacteria and fungi. Store the respirator in a cool, dry area.
- Protect the respirator from damage so that it maintains its shape and fit to
  your face. A damaged or misshapen respirator can leak.

Respirators must be worn when in close proximity with a patient who is suspected of having tuberculosis. EMS personnel must wear a respirator in the following situations:

- When entering the room of a person who may or does have tuberculosis.
- When performing invasive procedures such as endotracheal intubation or tracheal suctioning on a patient who has or is suspected of having tuberculosis.
- When transporting a tuberculosis patient in a closed vehicle.

When transporting a patient with tuberculosis, consider placing a surgical mask on the patient. This will reduce the amount of droplet material put into the air when the patient coughs and lower the risk of contamination of the equipment inside the vehicle. Be sure to monitor the patient's airway and breathing.

If the patient with tuberculosis is not breathing or assisted breathing is needed, a filter can be used with the bag-valve-mask device that reduces the risk of exposure to tuberculosis. A new device on the market consists of a fil-

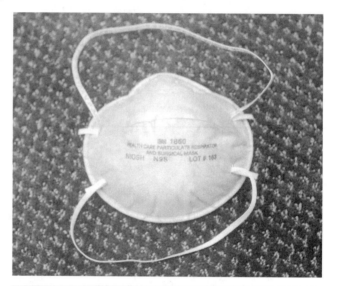

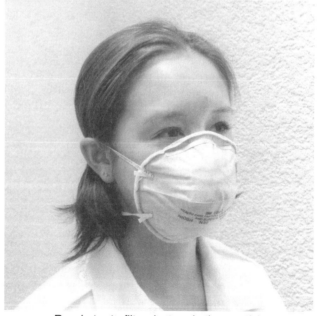

Respirator to filter dust and other particles.

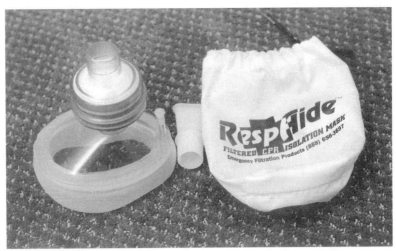

RespAide™ has filter to remove dust and other particles.

ter that fits the bag-valve-mask device and the resuscitation mask. As a single-use device, this filter will trap particulate matter and reduce possible contamination from the patient's airways and mucous membranes. The RespAide™ comes packaged as a kit containing the filter and face mask (see photo above). The kit also contains a mouthpiece that allows the device to be used in a personal first aid kit when a bag-valve-mask device is not available.

Gown or Protective Suit

A gown or protective suit should be worn whenever at risk for contamination of clothing. The type of gown or suit worn will depend on the situation. In most cases, a simple disposable gown will offer adequate protection. In extreme cases, you may want to wear a water-repellent gown or plastic apron over your gown. Jumpsuits or protective suits made of Tyvek® will meet this requirement. Many uniform or supply vendors have specially treated garments that repel moisture, some of which are disposable.

TRAINING PROGRAMS

The Bloodborne Pathogens Standard requires that the employer provide training in bloodborne pathogens at no cost to the employee and during normal working hours. This training must be provided when initially assigned to a job with a potential for exposure to bloodborne pathogens. For most EMTs and paramedics, this means the time they are hired.

In addition to the initial training in bloodborne pathogens, the employer must conduct annual training programs plus inservice programs whenever there are changes in the Infection Control Program.

Not only does OSHA's Bloodborne Pathogen Standard require comprehensive training in bloodborne diseases, but the CDC's Tuberculosis Control Program also requires training in tuberculosis control and prevention. If the two sets of guidelines are combined, a thorough educational program can be developed.

The training program must include the following components:

- The contents of the Bloodborne Pathogens Standard. It is not necessary to provide a copy to each employee; however, the employee does have the right to review a copy of the Standard.

- The nature, spread, signs, and symptoms of bloodborne pathogens and tuberculosis.
- The methods of transmitting bloodborne and airborne pathogens to identify risks of exposure.
- The employer's exposure control plan and copies of the written plan.
- How to recognize parts of the job that put the employee at risk for exposure to blood and other infectious agents.
- The methods used to reduce exposure along with their limitations. This shall also include a discussion on engineering controls, work practices, and personal protective equipment.
- How to handle and dispose of contaminated personal protective equipment.
- Information on the hepatitis B vaccine along with the safety, efficacy, and method of administration of the vaccine. The vaccination will be provided at no cost to the employee.
- The procedures to follow when exposed, including how to report the incident and the follow-up procedures involved, including blood or skin testing.

The employer must keep records of all training. These records must include the dates of the training, the contents or summary of the training session, the names and qualifications of the instructor(s), and the names and job titles of everyone attending the program. This information must remain on file for a minimum of three years from the date of the training and be available to the employee as well as any representative from the Department of Labor or OSHA.

VACCINATIONS AGAINST HEPATITIS B

The employer must offer the hepatitis B vaccination series within 10 working days after being assigned to a high-risk position. In EMS, this generally means within 10 days after the start of employment. There is no cost to the employee for the vaccination series.

There are occasions when the vaccination may not be administered. This occurs when:

- The vaccination series has already been received.
- Testing indicates an immunity to hepatitis B virus.
- Vaccination is contraindicated for medical reasons such as allergy to the vaccination serum.
- The employee declines to be vaccinated. An employee can refuse to be vaccinated but can change his or her mind at a later date. If choosing to accept the vaccination later, the employer must make it available.

The series of vaccinations includes three intramuscular injections. After the initial injection, a second vaccination is administered in 30 days. The third injection is given at 6 months. Occasionally, a booster vaccination may be required. The employer is also required to make the booster available at no cost. The employer is required to maintain a record of immunizations or refusals to be immunized.

In addition to the hepatitis B vaccination, other vaccinations may be made available. Such vaccinations include measles, mumps, and rubella as well as chickenpox and hepatitis A. To date, there is no standard requiring employers to offer these immunizations. If concerned about the other immunizations, contact your physician and ask about their availability.

LABELING AND HANDLING INFECTIOUS WASTE

Infectious waste and contaminated disposable items must be properly handled to prevent risk of accidental exposure. OSHA requires that soiled items be placed in a specially labeled container for biohazards and disposed of properly. For disposable sharps, a red, tamperproof plastic container is to be provided. The employer is responsible for disposing of the filled container in accordance with federal, state, and local laws. It is the EMT or paramedic's responsibility to use the container properly and let the supervisor or Infec-tion Control Officer know when the container is full and needs to be replaced.

Most EMS agencies are using disposable linens for the gurneys. Some agencies still use washable linens. In cold climates, blankets may be used to protect patients from extremes in temperature. These items will become contaminated with blood or infectious agents. If laundry is soiled, place it in a red biohazard bag and transport it to an approved location for cleaning. If there is a chance that the bag could leak, place it in a leak-proof container. Wear gloves and appropriate personal protective equipment when handling soiled laundry (see photo below).

POSTEXPOSURE PROCEDURES

Even with all the protections in place, accidental exposure may occur. Part of the Infection Control Plan is to provide comprehensive postexposure procedures to ensure the employee's health and treatment. If exposed to an infec-

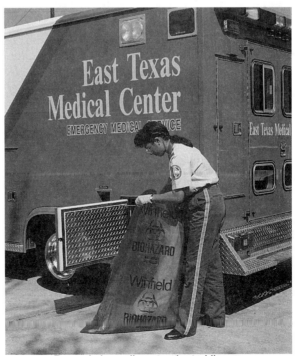

Properly bag all contaminated linens.

tious agent including HIV, HBV, or tuberculosis, report the exposure to the supervisor or Infection Control Officer immediately. The employer must, according to OSHA standards, provide a confidential medical examination that includes, at a minimum:

- Route(s) and circumstances of exposure.
- Identification of the source individual, unless this is not feasible or not possible under current state or local laws. The employee may have some rights under the Ryan White CARE Act to obtain information concerning the source individual.
- Testing and results of the source individual's blood. Consent for testing must be obtained from the source individual and, if it cannot be obtained, the employer must document refused consent. If consent is not necessary, the source individual's blood will be tested and the results documented.
- The results of the test will be made available to the employee.

The employer is responsible not only for obtaining the above information but also for maintaining postexposure medical records. These records are considered confidential and cannot be shared with anyone without written permission. The medical record is required to contain, at a minimum:

- The employee's name and social security number
- Hepatitis B vaccination status
- Copies of results of medical examinations, tests results, and follow-up procedures
- Employer's copy of the health-care worker's written opinion

These records must be maintained while you are employed with that agency plus 30 years.

SUMMARY

This chapter has focused on the requirements established by the CDC and OSHA to implement an Infection Control Program to protect employees' health and safety while working. The employer is required to provide equipment and the means to reduce accidental exposure to bloodborne pathogens and tuberculosis.

The employer is responsible for providing training in bloodborne pathogens as well as tuberculosis, vaccinations against hepatitis B, personal protective equipment, and procedures to follow in the event of an accidental exposure. The employer is also responsible for establishing workplace safety including policies and procedures to reduce risk for exposure.

The EMT or paramedic has a responsibility in assuring safety by following the guidelines established by the CDC, OSHA, and his or her employer. Health and safety are everyone's responsibility.

Appendix
Example of a Written Infection Control Program

INFECTION CONTROL PROGRAM

As an employee with ABC EMS Agency, the risk of infection and subsequent illness each time an employee is exposed to blood or potentially infectious materials is great. The Infection Control Program (ICP) is the core element used to reduce the risk by minimizing or eliminating exposure incidents to bloodborne pathogens such as HBV and HIV. This ICP is the company's oral and written policy relating to the control of infectious disease hazards.

Exposure Determination

The following positions associated with employment have been determined to have a degree of risk to exposure.

Position	Degree of Risk
Ambulance and EMS personnel	High
Office personnel	Low
Vehicle maintenance personnel	Low

Control Methods—Universal Precautions

The term *universal precautions* refers to a method of infection control in which blood and other potentially infectious materials are handled as if known to be infectious for HBV or HIV. Universal precautions apply to everything including blood, feces, urine, mucus secretions, vomit, and more, even if blood is not visible.

Control Methods—Work Practice Controls

Work practice controls are defined as alterations in the manner in which a task is performed in an effort to reduce the likelihood of an employee's exposure to blood or potentially infectious materials.

Hands will be washed with soap and water after removing gloves or as soon as possible following contact with body fluids.

All personal protective equipment will be removed immediately, or as soon as possible upon leaving the work area, and placed in an appropriately

105

designated area or container for storage, washing, decontamination, or disposal.

All procedures involving blood or other potentially infectious materials will be performed in such a manner as to minimize splashing and spraying.

Personal Protective Equipment

Personal protective equipment is defined as specialized clothing or equipment used by workers to protect themselves from direct exposure to blood or other potentially infectious materials.

The company will provide and assure employee use of appropriate personal protective equipment such as, but not limited to, gloves, gowns, face masks, protective goggles, resuscitation bags, pocket masks, or other ventilation devices when there is a potential for exposure to blood or other potentially infectious materials. Such equipment shall be readily accessible and available in the appropriate sizes.

The company will provide for cleaning, laundering, and disposal of protective equipment. The company will also repair or replace protective equipment as needed to maintain its effectiveness.

Surgical or examination gloves will be replaced when visibly soiled, torn, punctured, or when their integrity is compromised. Surgical or examination gloves will not be washed nor disinfected for reuse.

HBV Vaccination

HBV vaccinations are offered at no cost to the EMS employee on a voluntary basis. The HBV vaccination consists of three inoculations with the second and third injections at one month and six months, respectively. Contact the Infection Control Officer for more information.

Postexposure Evaluation and Follow-Up

After receiving a report of an exposure incident, the company will make available to the employee a confidential medical evaluation and follow-up of the incident. The company will document the route of exposure, HBV, HIV, or TB status of the patient(s) if known, and the circumstances under which the exposure occurred.

The company will notify the source patient(s) of the incident and attempt to obtain consent to collect and test the source blood for the presence of HBV and/or HIV. Further, the company will offer to collect a blood sample from the exposed employee as soon as possible after the exposure to determine HIV and HBV status. ABC EMS Agency will offer repeat HIV testing to exposed employees 6 weeks postexposure and on a periodic basis thereafter (at 12 weeks and again 6 months after exposure). Skin testing for tuberculosis will also be provided.

Follow-up of the exposed employee shall include counseling, the medical evaluation of any acute febrile illness that occurs with 12 weeks postexposure, and the use of safe and effective postexposure measures according to recommendations for standard medical practice.

Infectious Waste Disposal

Disposal of all infectious waste shall be in accordance with applicable federal, state, and local regulation. All infectious waste shall be disposed of by utilizing the hospital's infectious waste containers. When this is not available, the infectious waste must be bagged in a leak-proof container or color-coded bag and then labeled or tagged.

If laundry is soiled, it must be placed in a ABC EMS Agency–approved waste disposal bag and then placed with the remainder of the laundry.

Tags, Labels, and Bags

Biohazards at ABC EMS Agency will be tagged and labeled as mandated under Article 29, CFR 1910.145 and will be used to identify the presence of an actual or potential hazard.

Decontamination

After each transport, the inside of the vehicle carrying a potentially infectious patient will be disinfected (see photo that follows). The employee will use the company-issued disinfectant wipes and/or spray and decontaminate all exposed surfaces as soon as possible prior to any subsequent call.

Initial cleanup of blood or other potentially infectious materials shall include cleaning the equipment with soap and water along with the use of an approved hospital disinfectant chemical germicide that is considered tuberculoidal or by using a solution of 5.25 sodium hypochlorite (household bleach) diluted in a 1:10 to 1:100 mixture with water.

All equipment contaminated with blood or potentially infectious materials will be checked and decontaminated prior to servicing or shipping.

Training and Education on Infectious Disease Policies

ABC EMS Agency shall ensure that all employees with exposure to blood or other potentially infectious materials participate in a training and education program. Material appropriate in content and vocabulary to the educational level, literacy, and language background of the employee will be used.

The following material will be covered in the new-employee orientation and on an as-needed basis with current employees. The training will be conducted on a one-on-one basis or in a group setting.

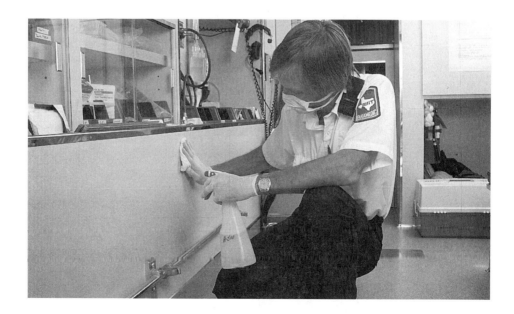

- An explanation of the epidemiology and signs and symptoms of HBV, HIV, and tuberculosis.
- An explanation of the mode of transmission of HBV, HIV, and tuberculosis.
- An explanation of the ABC EMS Agency Infection Control Program.
- An explanation of the use and limitations of methods of control that may prevent or reduce exposure. These include universal precautions, engineering controls, work practices, and personal protective equipment.
- An explanation of the basis for selection of personnel protective equipment.
- Information on the HBV vaccine, including its efficacy, safety, and the benefits of being vaccinated.
- An explanation of the procedures following an exposure, method of reporting the incident, and the medical follow-up that will be made available.

Record Keeping

The company shall track each worker's reported exposure. In the event of exposure to HBV or HIV, the incident will be recorded on the OSHA 200 log if the illness can be traced to an injury or other exposure incident.

Below are sample forms for use in an Infection Control Program. The forms can be modified to fit individual agency requirements.

ABC EMS Agency
Personal Protection Equipment
Mandated by OSHA Bloodborne Pathogens Standard

Required Personal Protective Equipment

Employee's Name _____ Date _____

Job Title _____

Primary Job Task _____

Equipment:

- ❑ Nonsterile medical gloves   ❑ Gown   ❑ Eye protection
- ❑ Utility gloves   ❑ Mask   ❑ Face protection
- ❑ CPR mouth-to-mouth barrier

_____

Signature of Health Professional Issuing Items

I hereby acknowledge that I have received the items checked above issued to me for my personal safety and protection.

_____

Signature of Employee

ABC EMS Agency
Training Session Form
Mandated by OSHA Bloodborne Pathogens Standard

To be completed for all training session participants

Employee's Name _____ Date _____

Job Title _____

Employee Identification Number _____

I have received training covering the following topics:

❑ Spread of HBV and HIV infection in the general population.

❑ Symptoms and effects of HBV and HIV infection.

❑ Ways of preventing, detecting, and treating HBV and HIV infections.

❑ How to deal with sexual partners of people with HBV and HIV infections and those at special risk of getting hepatitis B or AIDS.

_____

Signature of Trainer

I hereby acknowledge that I have received training in the items checked above.

_____

Signature of Employee

ABC EMS Agency
Hepatitis B Vaccination
Statement Declining Vaccine
Mandated by OSHA Bloodborne Pathogens Standard

Please read the information below and sign this statement indicating that you are declining the voluntary vaccination against hepatitis B.

I understand that, due to my occupational exposure to blood or potentially infectious materials, I may be at risk of acquiring hepatitis B (HBV) infection. I have been given the opportunity to be vaccinated with hepatitis B vaccine at no charge to me.

However, I **decline** hepatitis B vaccination at this time. I understand that by declining this vaccine, I continue to be at risk of acquiring hepatitis B, a serious disease.

If, in the future, I continue to have occupational exposure to blood or other potentially infectious materials and I want to be vaccinated with hepatitis B vaccine, I can receive the vaccination series at no charge to me.

_____

Signature of Employee

_____

Date Signed

ABC EMS Agency
Hepatitis B Vaccination
Documentation Form
Mandated by OSHA Bloodborne Pathogens Standard

Employee's Name _____

Employee Identification Number _____

HBV Vaccination Record

Series	Date	Administered By	Lot #

Vaccine 1

Vaccine 2

Vaccine 3

_____
Signature of Employee

You Make the Call
Answers

CHAPTER 1—INTRODUCTION

The man in this situation seems to be intoxicated and is probably vomiting because of excessive drinking. The vomiting is probably not an indication of an infectious disease—but you cannot absolutely rule out other causes of his vomiting. You should wear gloves when evaluating and treating this patient. Emesis could contain some hidden blood or be harboring bacteria from food poisoning. Universal precautions are essential to protect against bloodborne or other infectious agents.

CHAPTER 2—MODES OF DISEASE TRANSMISSION

The man may have an upper respiratory infection from the flu or he could have pneumonia from a secondary bacterial infection. In either case, he should be considered infectious. The disease may be contracted by droplet infection or by indirect contact. When the man coughs, contaminated droplets of moisture from his airways are expelled into the air. These droplets can be introduced into the body if inhaled. Infection could also occur by indirect contact. When the man coughs infectious sputum and discards the sputum in a tissue, the tissue is infectious. Touching or picking up any misplaced tissues could bring the viruses or bacteria into contact with the skin. From there, the organisms could be introduced into the body by rubbing the eyes, eating, or using contaminated eating utensils before washing the hands. Although direct contact is another means of transmitting infectious diseases, in this situation, direct contact is unlikely.

Protect against unwanted exposure by wearing gloves. If the man is coughing copious amounts of mucus, a mask and eye protection are appropriate. After completing the call, wash hands thoroughly before eating or drinking.

A flu shot will not offer complete protection against the flu. The immunization will protect against the strains of influenza known at the time the vaccine was developed. However, a new strain of influenza could still cause infection.

CHAPTER 3—THE IMMUNE SYSTEM

The body has several defense mechanisms to protect against contracting an infectious disease. In the example given, there are several reasons why illness did not occur when exposed to the cold or flu virus. First, the natural barriers or natural defenses offered protection. Second, the immune system prevented the viruses from invading the body and causing disease.

The natural barriers include the skin and the linings of the airways and organ systems that may come in contact with the organisms. These natural barriers prevent an infection from gaining access to the body.

The immune system also acts to protect by a process known as phagocytosis. If some of the organisms manage to survive these defenses, the immune system, with its antibodies and specialized lymphocytes, will prevent infection. Antibodies allow the body's immune system to immediately recognize an invading organism and stimulate the immune system to act.

It is not necessary to wear a surgical mask during cold and flu season to protect against the illnesses. The body's natural resistance will provide protection. If advised, get a flu shot at the beginning of the flu season.

CHAPTER 4—COMMUNICABLE DISEASES OF CHILDHOOD

The most likely cause of the girl's complaint is epiglottitis, a bacterial infection causing an inflamed and swollen epiglottis. It is essential that the child's throat not be examined because direct visualization of the epiglottis could result in a complete obstruction of the airway.

Because the infectious agent is bacterial and is located in the upper airway, it can be spread by droplet infection as well as direct contact. Even though the condition is rarely seen in adults, universal precautions should be taken.

The second case involves a child with chickenpox. If chickenpox was contracted as a child, there is an acquired immunity to the virus. A vaccination is also available for those who did not have the disease as a child. Without the vaccination, contracting the illness is possible. Using universal precautions will reduce the chance of exposure.

CHAPTER 5—INFECTIOUS DISEASES FOUND IN ADULTS

Based upon the information given, suspect tuberculosis. Immediately don protective face masks including the HEPA mask or approved nonporous mask in addition to gloves. If appropriate and patient care will not be compromised, have the patient also wear a nonporous mask. Promptly isolating the patient from family members or other crew members is important.

Remember that tuberculosis can be spread easily by dried droplets. Prior to transporting the man to the hospital, have unnecessary equipment removed from your vehicle if at all feasible. A supervisor's vehicle or another ambulance may be able to assist in this task. Otherwise, protect the equipment from contamination by covering it as much as possible. While en route to the hospital, use the patient compartment exhaust fan to help remove infected particles from the ambulance. After turning the patient over to the hospital staff, thoroughly disinfect the ambulance with a cleaning agent labeled to destroy tuberculosis bacteria.

After transporting a tuberculosis patient, consider a PPD skin test to determine exposure. If the test is positive, a chest X-ray and prophylactic antibiotic treatment may be ordered.

CHAPTER 6—FOOD POISONING

In the case study, the most likely cause of the food poisoning is *Escherichia coli.* Unpasteurized fruit juices or milk as well as beef products can contain the bacteria that cause this severe form of food poisoning. In addition to *E. coli,* other bacteria such as salmonella and staphylococcus can lead to food poisoning. Salmonella bacteria are typically found in raw chicken or eggs whereas staphylococcus bacteria are found in tainted dairy products.

At home, use reasonable precautions when handling food. When handling raw chicken, eggs, or beef, be sure to wash hands thoroughly after touching the foods. Also, clean any surfaces such as cutting boards that the raw foods may have contacted before using again. Completely cook these foods because cooking destroys the bacteria.

CHAPTER 7—HIV AND AIDS

Although not all AIDS patients exhibit all of the signs and symptoms, be aware of the major findings associated with the disease. The patient in the case study presented with a sufficient number of signs and symptoms to suspect HIV or AIDS.

Because of the body's weakened immune system, opportunistic infections can develop. A likely cause of the man's difficulty breathing is *pneumocystis carinii* pneumonia whereas another opportunistic infection could be the cause of the man's trouble swallowing. Candidiasis or oral thrush extending into the throat can cause pain when swallowing.

When providing care for this patient, universal precautions are in order and will depend upon the nature of the treatment to be provided. At a minimum, gloves shall be worn. A mask and goggles with or without a gown might be appropriate if splashing with body fluids is possible.

CHAPTER 8—HEPATITIS—AN ALPHABET SOUP

Hepatitis C can be much easier to transmit than HIV. Even dried blood should be considered infectious. In caring for the man in the case presented, wear gloves and, if splashing of blood if possible, wear a face mask, goggles, and gown. Any contaminated dressings or clothing should be discarded in appropriately labeled containers.

The dried blood on the cabinet found after the call should be considered highly infectious because current research shows that it can cause infection for up to three weeks. Clean the surface of the cabinet with disinfectant approved for use against hepatitis C. Wiping the cabinet with alcohol will not be acceptable.

Index

Abdominal pains, 10
Acquired immunity, 22–23
Acquired immunodeficiency syndrome (AIDS). *See* HIV and AIDS
Adult infectious diseases, 44–60
Agents, infectious, 2, 6
 types of, 7–8
Agglutination, 19, 23
AIDS. *See* HIV and AIDS
Airborne infections, 13, 14–15
Animal bites, 15
Anorexia, 70
Antibiotics, 56–58
Antibodies, 19, 22–23
Antigens, 19, 23
Antitoxins, 62
Asymptomatic, 45, 79
 HIV infection, 70, 73
Asymptomatic meningitis, 45

Babinski's reflex, 45, 49–50
Bacteria, 2, 7, 8
Bites, animal, 15
Bloodborne Pathogens Standard, 4–5, 86, 101–2
Blood transfusions, 15
B-lymphocytes, 19, 22–23
Botulism, 66, 68

***Candida albicans*, 70, 74, 75**
Candidiasis, 70, 73, 75
Centers for Disease Control and Prevention (CDC), 3–4, 86–87
 classification of AIDS, 73–74
 mission statement, 3–4
 Tuberculosis Control Program, 5
Chancres, 45
Chickenpox, 28–29, 42
Childhood diseases, 26–43
Chills, 10
Chlamydia, 54–55, 60
Chlamydia trachomitis, 55
Cilia, 19, 21
Cirrhosis, 79
Clostridium botulinum, 62, 66

Co-infections, 79
Complement system, 23
Conjunctivitis, 27, 36, 43
Contagious, 13
Contaminated surfaces, 15
Control plan. *See* Infection Control Plan
Coughing, 9, 14–15
Counseling, 5
Crepitus, 45
Croup, 27, 32, 42
Cryptosporidium enterocolitis, 70, 75
Cryptosporidosis, 70
Cyanosis, 27
Cytomegalovirus, 70, 73–75

Debridment, 45
Decontamination, 93–94, 107
Defenses of body, 19–25
Delta hepatitis (hepatitis D), 81
Diarrhea, 9
Diphtheria, 27, 35–36, 43
Direct contact, 15
Disease transmission modes, 7, 13–17
Disinfection, 86, 90, 93–94
Droplet infection, 13
Drug-resistant bacteria, 56–58
Dustborne infections, 13
Dysphagia, 27
Dyspnea, 27

***E. coli,* 62, 64–65, 68, 115**
Employee's role, 6
Encephalitis, 45
Encephalopathy, 27, 70
Engineering controls, 4, 86, 87–90
Enteric infections, 79–81
Enterococcus, 57–58
Enterohemorrhagic, 62, 64
Entry, portal of, 7, 13
Epidemic parotitis, 31–32
Epiglottitis, 27, 32–33, 42, 48–49, 59
Escherichia coli, 62, 64–65, 68, 115
Exit, portal of, 7
Exposure, 2, 4, 13